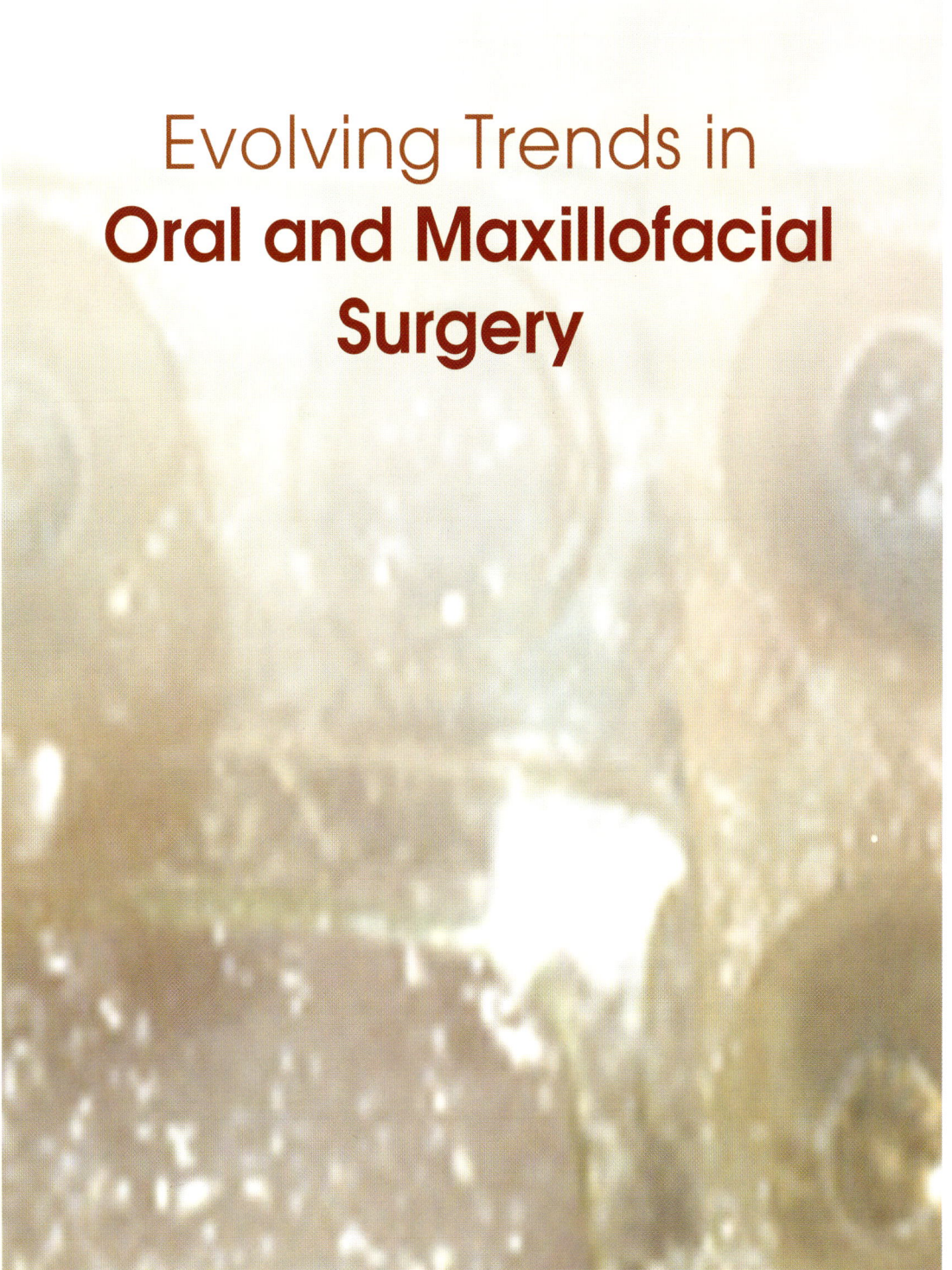

Evolving Trends in
Oral and Maxillofacial
Surgery

To be conscious of your own ignorance is the first step towards education

. …. Anonymous

Salient Features of the Book

- Excellent review of the historic development of dentistry.
- Wide and interesting text of evolution of oral and maxillofacial surgery as a speciality.
- Well illustrated text with drawings, diagrams and clinical photographs.
- Simple, lucid and understandable language and text.
- Concise information of current surgical principles and procedures.
- Precise coverage of latest revolutionary advances and techniques and future scope in oral and maxillofacial surgery.

Evolving Trends in
Oral and Maxillofacial Surgery

CHANDRAKANT P. TAWARE BDS, MDS (Bombay)

—

Honorary Professor and Postgraduate Teacher
University of Bombay

—

Department of Oral and Maxillofacial Surgery
Government Dental College and Hospital, Mumbai

—

Joint Director (Dental), Directorate of Medical Education and
Research (DMER), Maharashtra

—

Ex-Dean, Government Dental College and Hospital, Mumbai

—

Ex-Director, Directorate of Medical Education and
Research (DMER), Maharashtra

—

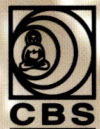

CBS

CBS Publishers & Distributors
New Delhi • Bangalore • Pune (India)

Evolving Trends in
**Oral and Maxillofacial
Surgery**

© 2009, Author and Publisher

First Edition 2009

ISBN: 978-81-239-1651-4

Published by Satish Kumar Jain and produced by Vinod K. Jain for
CBS Publishers & Distributors,
CBS Plaza, 4819/XI, Prahlad Street, 24 Daryaganj, New Delhi 110 002
E-mail: cbspubs@vsnl.com; cbspubs@airtelmail.in • Website: www.cbspd.com

Branch Offices:

• Seema House, 2975, 17th Cross, K.R. Road, Banasankari 2nd Stage, Bangalore 70
  Fax : 080-26771680 • E-mail : cbsbng@vsnl.net

• Shaan Brahmha Complex, Basement, Appa Balwant Chowk, Budhwar Peth,
  Next to Ratan Talkies, Pune 411002
  Fax : 020-24464059 • E-mail : pune@cbspd.com

Printed at:
Ajanta Offset and Packagings Ltd.

to

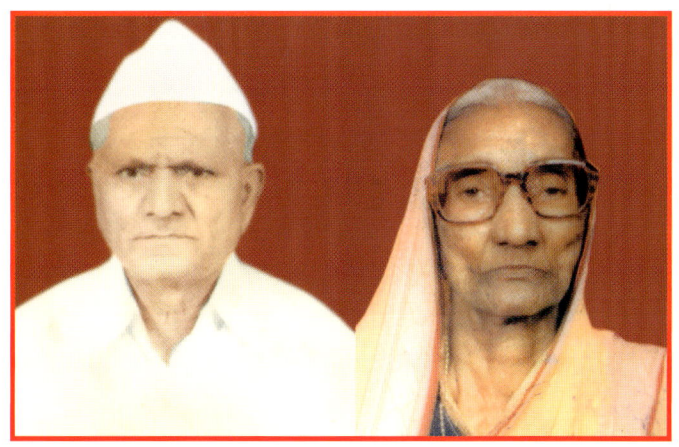

my parents

Late Shri Pandurang
and
Smt Bhagirathi Taware

who nurtured and cared for me
in true sense

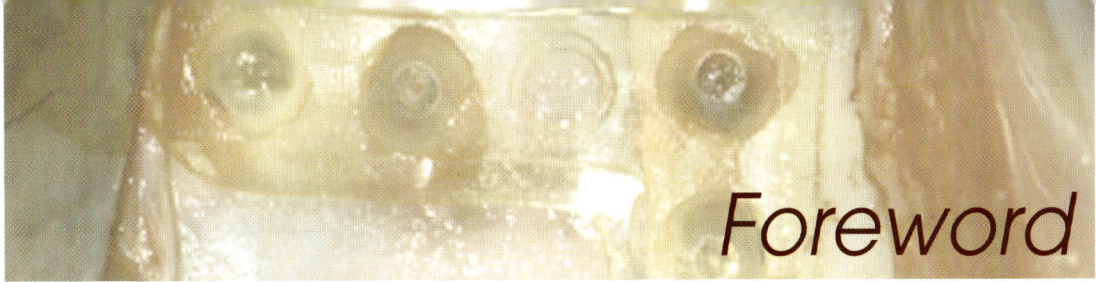

Foreword

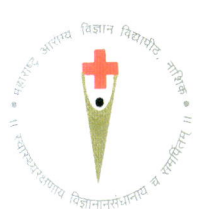

महाराष्ट्र आरोग्य विज्ञान विद्यापीठ, नाशिक
Maharashtra University of Health Sciences, Nashik
वणी-दिंडोरी रोड, म्हसरूळ, नाशिक-४२२००४., Vani-Dindori Road, Mhasrul, Nashik-422004

Tel : (0253) 2531835, Fax : (0253) 2539113. Mumbai (off.) Tele Fax : (022) 22653543
Website: www.muhsnashik.com   email: vc@muhsnashik.com/ muhsvc@hotmail.com

It gives me immense pleasure to write this Foreword to the book *Evolving Trends in Oral and Maxillofacial Surgery* written by Dr. Chandrakant. P. Taware. It is said: "To understand our roots is to better gauge and appreciate the present professional position. Looking back can prevent misunderstanding and false assumptions, and that look can bring the wisdom needed to face the challenges of our future mission in health care."

Dr. Taware has held a number of posts during his academic career and has tremendous experience in every walk of life. He has been the postgraduate teacher for a number of students. He has held offices as Joint Director as well as the Director for the State of Maharashtra.

This book provides a glimpse of how dentistry was practised in the past and how oral and maxillofacial surgery developed as a specialised branch of dentistry. History always remains a mystery till one becomes aware of it and Dr. Taware has made sincere efforts to help his comrades and the professionals unfold that mystery. The book provides comprehensive information on how dentistry was practised in the stone-age and how it has evolved to the present situation. The author has done a noble job of acknowledging the efforts made by the personnel in helping the profession reach this day from the stone-age.

"Just like a stream, the beginning of all big things are small" and I believe this effort made by Dr. Taware will enlighten us all. I wish this book a great success and believe that the professionals would await subsequent editions of this book.

Dr (Mrs) Mrudula A. Phadke
Vice-Chancellor
Maharashtra University of Health Sciences, Nashik

Preface

Change is the only continuum …

L ife is ever changing and with changing times it changes its colours and style. Life requirements are ever changing, hence pertaining efforts to achieve goals are also ever changing. It equally and universally applies to all concepts. It is a well known fact that concepts today were not exactly the same as in the nearest past or say the last decade, century and or in the ancient times. It happened in every walk of human life since the primitive era. It has happened in the same way in dentistry today.

Dental profession and dental health care system today have acquired tremendous importance in human life across the globe. Indeed it is a fact that in all developed countries the dental profession has reached its peak in all aspects and it is being followed on the same footprints in the developing countries. With acquisition of newer concepts, continuous research in biological fields, improving applications of latest technological know-how to health care systems, every aspect of dentistry is continuously evolving and getting more advanced and refined — right from diagnosis to treatment aspects.

Oral and maxillofacial surgery is an indispensable speciality of dentistry which too has evolved from simply being science of extraction of tooth to dentoalveolar surgery, oral surgery involving surgery of jaws apparatus, and to its present form which deals with the entire facial structure and associated maladies. Even this is fast becoming more and more sophisticated, broader and wider, as it is taking many steps further into various fields like minimally invasive aesthetic facial surgery, oral cancer surgery, skull base surgery and craniomaxillofacial surgery, thus galloping at a great pace.

Rome was not built in a day. You cannot build a magnificent structure without a solid, strong foundation. It is our moral duty as oral and maxillofacial surgeons and dental specialists to know what our roots are. How did it all begin? What brought us where we are now? Someone has rightly said: "The good deeds of great men never go waste, because the history of the world is an autobiography of these great men."

From the darkness of superstitions, myths, false-believes which once influenced human treatment practices, it was the work of a few determined pioneers, often working alone, who dedicatedly assembled their knowledge and experiences in some scientific order. With efforts of these individuals and teachers who devoted their professional careers to this field, toiled, applied innovative concepts, taught and inspired their students, our comprehension of all modalities of treating human ailments has, and is, accumulating at logarithmic speed. Research, utilization and application of advances in other areas of science has contributed significantly to recent knowledge. The practice of oral and maxillofacial surgery today is far more efficient, reliable and advanced from what it was initially at its emergence as a specialty.

It has been my sincere wish from many years to come up with some work which lightens this evolution of my specialty which is ever-changing. This book is my humble and honest effort in a lucid, interesting and understanding language as an attempt to highlight progressive changes in practice of oral and maxillofacial surgery to its present form and promises it has to offer in future.

Now giving a brief introduction of this work, the first two chapters introduce various practices of dentistry from a primitive era where different concepts and methods were followed for oral and dental health care in various civilizations at different times across the globe, and how the practice of dentistry started shaping up into a more scientific and biological one. In the third and fourth chapters, information is given specifically about the historic development of oral surgery as a specialty and a brief outlook of various surgical procedures and protocols followed in modern practice of oral and maxillofacial surgery, dealing with dentoalveolar surgery, facial trauma surgery, orthognathic surgery, temporomandibular joint surgery, cleft lip and palate surgery and oral cancer surgery, etc. The fifth chapter describes the current scenario of newer practices being introduced in oral and maxillofacial surgery like lasers, cryosurgery, gene therapy, craniomaxillofacial surgery and the latest trends which advocate minimally invasive, less morbid, more preservative surgical principles and better postsurgical outcomes for the patients. The sixth chapter describes the future scope and promises the specialty has in offering, to reach newer heights.

I really consider myself fortunate to witness this all in my speciality and I am amazed to see how rapidly it has progressed into a more principled, scientific and patient-friendly practice. My love, belief and dedication in my specialty has become more solid and stronger and this has been instrumental to inspire me to work and to put up with this endeavour. I strongly believe that the speciality alongwith the other biomedical sciences, especially those which are dedicated to health care system, is ever-changing, ever-updating, ever-refining and ever-progressing. In the present presentation if any lacunae are left, which I do accept as my unawareness, I would be open for correction. I would love to accept suggestions which I feel are most valuable. Citations and figures depicting various transitions of dentistry and oral and maxillofacial surgery are being taken up as a courtesy, as mentioned in the bibliography.

I hope this book benefits the students, who are the core of educational system and the messengers for the excellence of the speciality. It will also be of good use for the teachers, the practitioners in the speciality of dentistry and oral and maxillofacial surgery, and even to the common man who wants to know about the subject in this regard.

Chandrakant P. Taware

Acknowledgements

I would like to thank Almighty for everything I could ever get and have achieved in life.

I am equally indebted to my parents, late Shri Pandurang and Smt Bhagirathi Taware, for their efforts in bringing me up and instilling right principles and values in me.

I would like to thank my wife and my children for standing by me with their endless love, support and inspiration.

I would like to thank all my teachers, especially my mentor Dr. J.N. Khanna, Dr. Dudhani, Dr. S.S. Khera, Dr. Wadkar, Dr. A.P. Chitre, Dr. Vandekar, Dr. Kali Kapadia and all my teacher colleagues for inspiring me over the years in this subject. I would like to thank all my postgraduate students who have always supported me, inspired me, and were of great help to me.

I must thank my postgraduate student and my assistant Dr. Abdul A. Khan, now working as a Lecturer in Department of Oral and Maxillofacial Surgery at Government Dental College, Aurangabad, who strived hard and helped me very sincerely to bring this work to completion. I also acknowledge the efforts put in by my other postgraduate students Dr. Samir D. Khaire, Dr. Sagar Vaishampayan, and also all the staff in the Department of Oral and Maxillofacial Surgery, Government Dental College, Mumbai.

I express my sincere thanks to all those sources for permitting us to use figures mentioned in references.

I thank CBS Publishers and Distributors, New Delhi, for their efforts and support to publish my book.

The most important are my patients, who allowed me to serve them over the years and enriched my knowledge and experience not only in the speciality but also in my life too.

Chandrakant P. Taware

Dr. Chandrakant P. Taware has been in academics since 1976, and has worked in various capacities at Government Dental College, Mumbai, and Government Dental College, Aurangabad (Maharashtra). He is a postgraduate teacher in the subject of oral and maxillofacial surgery under Mumbai University, since 1991. He has been Professor and Head, Department of Oral and Maxillofacial Surgery, and Dean at Government Dental College, Mumbai. He was Director, Directorate of Medical Education and Research, Government of Maharashtra, Mumbai (Jan 2003–June 2004). He has been working as Joint Director (Dental), Directorate of Medical Education and Research (DMER), Maharashtra, since 2001.

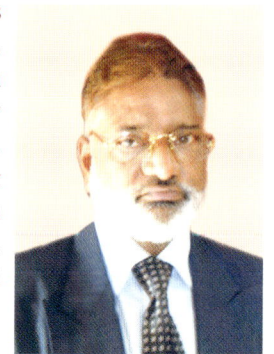

Dr. Taware has been examiner for undergraduate, postgraduate and DNB courses in the subject of oral and maxillofacial surgery, for Mumbai University and various universities across India. He has worked as ex-officio member of various advisory committees for Mumbai University and Maharashtra University of Health Sciences (MUHS), Maharashtra State Dental Council, and Dental Council of India in the capacities of Professor and Head, Dean, Joint Director and Director (DMER). He has presented many research papers at various state and national conferences. Besides these, he has made contributions to many national and international publications. He is truly a seasoned teacher, academician and administrator.

Contents

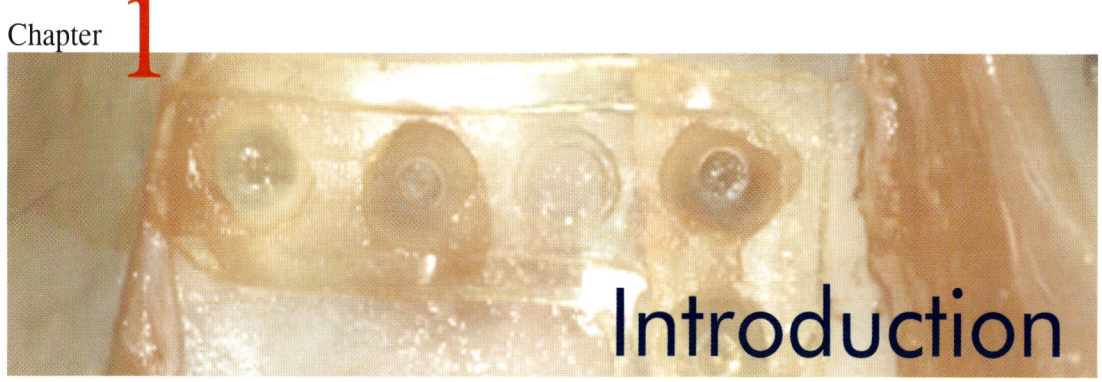

Chapter 1

Introduction

"Whoever wishes to foresee the future must consult the past; for human events ever resemble those of preceding times. This arises from the fact that they are produced by men who ever have been, and ever shall be, animated by the same passions, and thus they necessarily have the same results".

—*Machiavelli.*

Man has always been subject to disease. We know that disease is as old as life itself, that medicine is as old as man, that necessity that has ever been the mother of invention must have early taught him to use some means for alleviation or cure; rough and uncouth perhaps but still in a measure answering his purpose.[1]

Without a proper background no history would be complete, and therefore in presenting a retrospect of dentistry as it existed prior to the periods under consideration, attention must be focused upon the many difficulties with which our early colleagues were confronted. It is not only necessary but also imperative to do so in order that the bright and clear light of progress may be more effectively seen, understood and appreciated. To fully comprehend our present professional position and to evaluate whatever advancement has been made, we must take into consideration our early heritage and we should have some knowledge of the conditions extant through the early ages.[2]

The beginning of a definite and a continuous history of the profession, which we now call dentistry, can be placed with certainty about the early part of the eighteenth century and is associated with the great name of "Pierre Fauchard", the founder of modern dentistry. Yet a glance at the earliest medical treatises readily indicates that dental practice is centuries old. Research has shown that even the materials such as gold and silver, which we use at present, must have found like employment in the practice of dentistry in remote days. Prosthetic pieces, skulls and teeth have been discovered to offer proof of the accomplishments of this early dentistry. Many instruments and simple appliances were devised which we now regard as definite applications of present day dental principles.[3]

The historians believe that the fair test of judging the standard of a profession is its literature. For our knowledge of the earliest data we are in the first instance dependant upon evidence accumulated by the archaeological research of the remains of prehistoric man and in the second instance to surviving specimens and documentary records of ancient times. During the period of primitive medicine and dentistry, literature was very meagre, for the artisans were not scholars and in their anxiety to guard the secrets of their crafts, they failed to leave behind them any record of the details of their methods.[4]

History has failed to record when and by whom dentistry was first practiced but there is sufficient proof that efforts in that direction were made by the early Europeans, the Arabians and perhaps even by the South American Indians. Those in the old world apparently interested themselves only in prosthesis namely, the supplying of missing teeth whilst the New world was interested in the operative phase that is restoring through artificial means the individual tooth itself.[5]

The history of medicine and the history of dentistry as a so-called pure science are so inextricably interwoven that the consideration of one inevitably involves that of the other. There were times when both were but a collection of vaguely described traditions. One however does find a gradual development of dentistry along with surgery, although surgery almost always precedes internal medicine. The ancient concepts of physiology and pathology are, for the most part, now considered as being curious illustrations of human errors and only a portion of anatomy and surgery of the ancient remains as an essential part of the foundation of the art of medicine as we know it today.[6]

The origin of dentistry is lost in the mists of antiquity. It is our desire through the aid of ancient records to penetrate the mist and to show that the practice of dental art is as old as that of medicine and so closely interwoven thereto that one finds it impossible to distinguish one from the other.[7] A study of evolution teaches us that a series of steps are required whereby a germ or a rudimentary part becomes an adult organism or a fully developed part and that a succession of changes is required by which something complex is developed from simple beginnings.

The ascendancy of the healing art of the oral structures to the profession of dentistry is the end of a long journey from the roots of civilization to the age of molecular biology. The odd, frustratingly slow, often inspiring history, in which dentistry recently reached the established and recognized status of an independent specialty of the healing profession, can be retraced parallel to that of medicine as the issue of the following consecutive epochs:

First there is paleontologic evidence of the suffering of our human ancestors from oral ills and the first attempts of treatments by healers and sorcerers. Then comes the era of a rising recognition of the pathologic conditions at the dawn of the medical sciences. Then followed the dark period of the quackery- pharmacologic and technical, tool making revolution that lasted short of a few exceptions of scientific pioneering upto the eighteenth century.

The ultimate raise to the free academic profession is due to the scientific acquisitions of prestigious physiologists. The creation of dental faculties is the corner stone of the elevation of dentistry to a free academic profession, a process, which in old world countries as well as in the developing nations is still under way.

The history of dentistry in ancient times cannot be traced separately, as it is interlinked with the development of medical science. Magic and religion, not mathematics and astronomy, were the mental products of the early civilizations. Useless magical acts were considered to be of prime importance. The priesthood was often rooted in these rites. In the magic-bound Egyptian and Babylonian civilizations, toothache was believed to be a sign of divine displeasure. Relief could be sought by incantations and prayers.[1]

The "worm in the tooth" theory for the cause of toothache was believed by primitive people in all parts of the world as late as the 20th century.[2]

People of early ages had odd beliefs concerning teeth. The Egyptians believed that the mouse was under the direct protection of the sun; therefore if one had a toothache the split body of a warm mouse was applied to the affected side. In India the cuspid of Buddha was enshrined in a famous temple (at Kandi) and prayed to in fertility rites. Prayers were offered up to saints for the relief of pain.[3]

Teeth were knocked out as a form of punishment among early people of the Mesopotamian period.[4] During the Islamic age, the compensation for a knocked out tooth was 5 camels, which was a twentieth of what was paid for the life of a man.[5] Such was the scenario of dentistry in the ancient civilization. These ancient beliefs in magic, folklore, prejudices and personal superstitions that hampered medicine, also impeded the progress of dentistry.

According to Fielding H Garrison (1870–1935) before the time of Hippocrates medicine was regarded simply as a branch of philosophy and only began to flourish during the Age of Pericles with its scientific advancement centered in the figure of Hippocrates (160–370 BC) who gave to Greek medicine a scientific spirit and its ethical ideals.[6] Hippocrates appreciated the importance of teeth. He accurately described the technique for reducing a fracture of the jaw and also for replacing a dislocated mandible. He was familiar with extraction forceps. He also stated decay as a putrefactive process instead of fermentative.[7]

The great Roman physician Celsus believed that general physical deterioration caused dental diseases. Galen also a Roman, considered the greatest physician since Hippocrates, was the first to recognize that a toothache could be pulpitis or a pericementitis.[8] He classified the teeth into centrals, cuspids and molars. The famous French surgeon Guy de Chauliac was the first to coin the term DENTIST.[9] Previously they were known as the Operators of teeth, The Kindharts, The toothdrawers, the experts for the teeth or even the barbers.[10]

Subsequently came the era of specialization wherein eight branches took birth from dentistry namely orthodontics, Oral surgery, periodontics, prosthodontics, pedodontics, public health, oral pathology and finally endodontics in chronological order.[11]

The specialty of Oral and maxillofacial surgery came into existence in 1918. At that time it was called Oral surgery and was related to dental procedures such as dental extractions and minor dental procedures, mostly intraoral. Since then it has evolved through the ages broadening its scope to include the whole of the face and neck (when it was called oral and maxillofacial surgery). The present age of oral and maxillofacial surgery encompasses within its scope the management of:

1. Temporomandibular joint disorders
2. Maxillofacial trauma
3. Preprosthetic surgery
4. Cysts and Tumors of orofacial region including Neoplasia
5. Salivary gland disorders
6. Orofacial clefts
7. Maxillary sinus pathologies
8. Orofacial and neck infections
9. Facial neuropathology
10. Growth disturbances in the jaws.

Recently it has also included the various cranial procedures (osteotomies and augmentations) involved in the surgical management of the various craniofacial syndromes such as craniofacial dysostosis, craniosynostoses, etc. modifying it to the present age Craniomaxillofacial surgery.

This piece of work is a humble effort to present dentistry, since antiquity, with all its myths and facts and the evolution of the primitive, agonizing oral surgery from its inception undergoing refinements all the way to the present age of oral and maxillofacial surgery with its broad scope and advances resulting in its consideration as a bliss to the entire mankind.

The sole objective of our effort is to gather the relevant pieces of information and put together into fluent reading the fascinating tale of man's attempts over millenaries to conquer and prevent oral pain and disease, which in turn gives us detailed information as with ages together how the growth and development of original concepts, simultaneously adopting new innovative technologies and methodologies, outsourcing older concepts that suited the prevailing circumstances and ran well in association with all aspects of science and technology globally worked for the welfare of mankind and gave a new dimension to oral and maxillofacial surgery.

REFERENCES AND BIBLIOGRAPHY

1. The History of Dentistry in South Africa 1652-1900 by Dr Vilma Grobler 3.
2. *Idem.*
3. History of Dentistry 2001 by Terry Wilwerding 3.
4. History of Dentistry 2001 by Terry Wilwerding 4.
5. History of Dentistry by Walter Hoffman-Axthelm, 1981, Chapter 7, 91.
6. Garrison Fielding H.: An introduction to the history of Medicine. Phila., 4th edition, 1929, 92.
7. History of Dentistry 2001 by Terry Wilwerding 4.
8. History of Dentistry 2001 by Terry Wilwerding 5.
9. History of Dentistry 2001 by Terry Wilwerding 6.
10. History of Dentistry by Weinburger Volume 1 Chapter 1, 4.
11. History of Dentistry 2001 by Terry Wilwerding 4.
12. History of Dentistry by Weinburger Volume 1 Chapter 1, 1.
13. History of Dentistry by Weinburger Volume 1 Chapter 1, 5.
14. History of Dentistry by Weinburger Volume 1 Chapter 1, 7.
15, 16. *Idem.*
17. History of Dentistry by Weinburger Volume 1 Chapter 1, 8.
18. History of Dentistry by Weinburger Volume 1 Chapter 1, 7.

Chapter 2

Dentistry Since Antiquity

At the beginning, life consisted of simple creatures of the sea, which consisted of masses of protoplasmic cells. By engulfing themselves around a desired morsel, they were able to absorb food. Later a slit developed, the forerunner of the oral cavity and great gut. Much later tentacles and feelers developed around this slit. The tentacles helped to carry the food to the slit, oral cavity and great gut. Then nature took the outer layer of skin and carried it inward to the oral cavity. This skin contained tentacles that were the forerunners of our teeth. These tentacles, also called shagreen, were calcified. Some of these sea creatures developed lungs and became amphibians. Some began to spend time on land. At first they crawled on their bellies, later they developed limbs and feet and arose from the ground. Faced with a new environment including a mixed diet, the creatures evolved into stronger animals made up of hard bone and tough muscle fiber. Originally three single tentacles fused and became tri-conodonts. These later changed into teeth very similar to the teeth of the Catarrhine Apes (who inhabited the earth about 40,000,000 years ago in the middle of the Tertiary Period). The descendants of these apes have the same dental formula as man.[19]

Dental ailments have remained remarkably similar throughout history. If we set the beginning of history at 4000 BC, toothaches can be traced to the earliest records. In the Egyptian manuscripts known as Eber's Papyri, which dates back to 3700 BC, dental maladies such as toothaches and sore gums are mentioned.[20]

The exact time that dental art made its appearance isn't known; however, there is ample proof of its existence among the civilizations of Egypt, Etruscans of Central Italy, Assyrians, China, etc. Since Dental History is such a broad field, a few of the highlights of dentistry will be mentioned in order of importance and chronology.[21]

THE EGYPTIAN AGE

The first known dentist was an Egyptian named Hesi-Re (3000 BC).[22] He was the chief toothist to the Pharaohs. He was also a physician, indicating an association between medicine and dentistry. The Eber's papyrus was written between 1700 and 1500 BC and contains material dating back as far as 3700 BC. The Papyrus Ebers contains references to diseases of the teeth, as well as prescriptions for substances such as olive oil, dates, onions, beans, and green lead, to be mixed and applied "against the throbbing of the bennut blisters in the teeth."[23]

In the 5th century BC. Herodotus, a historian, described the medical art in Egypt: "The art of medicine is distributed thus: Each physician is a physician of one disease and no more; and the whole country is full of physicians, for some profess themselves to be physicians of the eyes, others of the head, others of the teeth, others of affections of the stomach, and others of more obscure ailments".[24] Much of early dentistry was practiced as part of the general practice of medicine.

Grapow believes that specialization as such did not exist in ancient Egypt, but that it appeared during the Egypt of Herodotus. However, he does recognize the man who deals with teeth for the ancient era.[25] The dental references found in papyrus scrolls, like the ophthalmologic and rhinological constituents of general therapy, are no proof of the existence of a speciality. Herodotus wrote that Egypt was full of specialists, enumerating the various parts of the body, including the teeth, treated by these so-called specialists. However, Egyptologists have been unable to find evidence of operative dental work in the wealth of well-preserved craniological material. The dry desert climate, together with the mummification process, perfected by the Egyptians with their keen sense of immortality, helped to preserve the ancient human remains. According to Dr. Campbell Thompson, the Assyriologist authority, the Edwin Smith surgical papyrus has no reference to dentistry.[26] Jones, a pathologist after examining numerous skeletons from the predynastic to the Christian and Coptic periods reported in 1910 that at no period do the teeth show signs of dentist's handiwork.[27] There is however, a description of a method to reduce a dislocated mandible.

The first evidence of a surgical operation was found in Egypt. A mandible with two perforations just below the root of the first molar indicated the establishment of drainage of an abscessed tooth. The approximate date is 2750 BC.

Egyptians also practiced the splinting of teeth as evidenced by a specimen from Gizeh, 2500 BC in which it shows two molars fastened with heavy gold wire.[28]

Early traces of preventive dentistry can be detected in two prescriptions

1. *The basic of a remedy for strengthening a tooth: Meal of a seed grain of emmer (a wheat-like flour)—1; ocher—1; honey—1. The mixture is to be pressed into a tooth.*

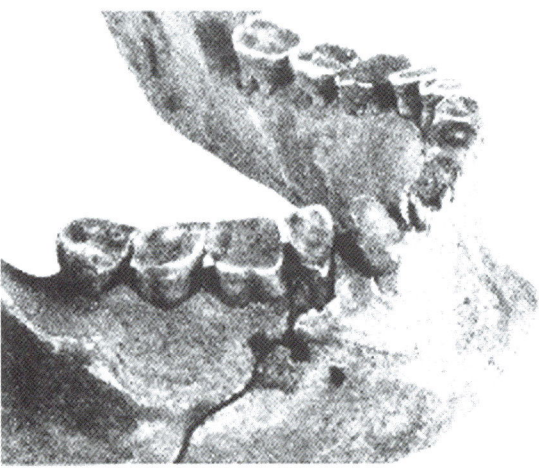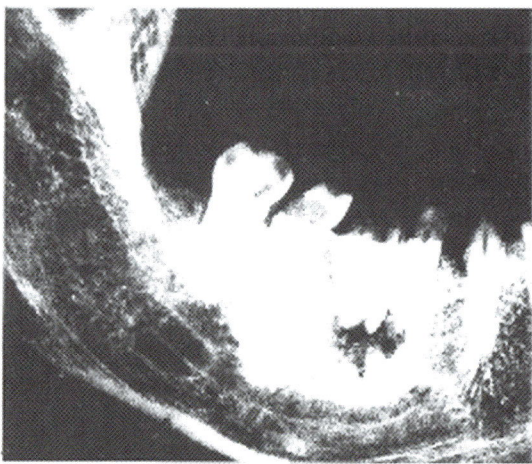

Fig. 2.1: Ancient Egyptian mandible (about 2500 BC) with questionable bore-holes and its radiograph.

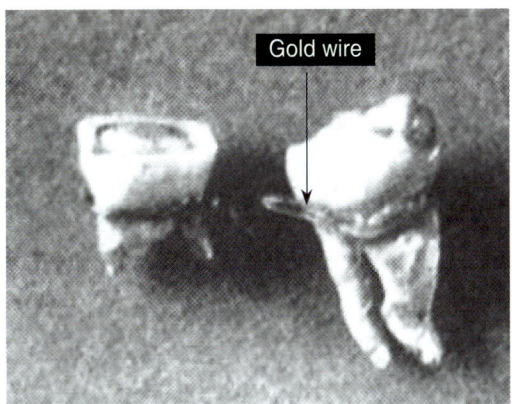

Fig. 2.2: Egyptian appliance found at Gizeh 2500 BC. Earliest known example of dental prosthesis, a gold wire woven around gingival margin of 3rd and 2nd left lower molars.

2. *Grinding stone powder—1; ocher—1; honey—1; this mixture is to be pressed into a tooth. Also a tooth powder for strengthening a tooth was prescribed: terebinthenic resin—1; ocher—1; malachite—1; the mixture is to be pulverized, to be applied to the tooth.*[29]

Quite contrary to today's standards was the advice to avoid all attempts at therapy for an infected jaw fracture. When you examine man with a fractured mandible, find the break with your hand as it is displaced beneath your fingers. In addition, if there is an open wound over the fracture and the discharge (?) has stopped flowing; he has fever as a consequence. This is a disease that cannot be treated.[30]

Newer (1973) radiographic examination of pharaoh mummies of the New Kingdom showed **no indication of tooth replacement.**[31]

THE CHINESE AGE

According to the history of the empire, Chinese medicine evolved in complete seclusion even from neighboring India until the 3rd century BC. Its beginnings were entirely different from those of earlier cultures whose medicine was mixed with religious ideas and at least in its early stage lay entirely in the hands of the priests and priest physicians. Chinese medicine was also intermingled with magical concepts.[32]

The Chinese were known to have treated dental ills with knife, cautery, and acupuncture, a technique whereby they punctured different areas of the body with a needle. There is no evidence of mechanical dentistry at that time, 2700 BC. Marco Polo stated that the Chinese did cover teeth with thin gold leafs only as decorations, 1280 AD.[33]

In the **GOLDEN MIRROR**, a gigantic encyclopedia begun at the close of the 18th century by the emperor's decree to collect historical and the most ancient knowledge, caries was designated as tooth worm traveling from one tooth to another. The first use of a toothbrush and of amalgam for cavity filling are attributed to Chinese medicine.[34]

THE MESOPOTAMIAN PERIOD

In Mesopotamia, Ashur-Bani-Pal ruled in Assyria 400 BC. He collected the store of Sumerian-Babylonian-Assyrian literature and science of two millennia in a giant clay tablet library. Numerous medical texts were found in the library of Ashurbanipal. Among these were

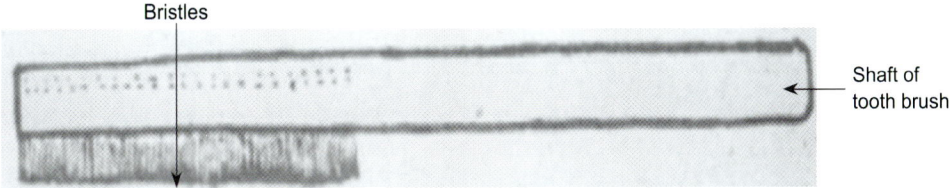

Fig. 2.3: The earliest known **modern toothbrush** stated to have been invented in **China.**

prescriptions for toothache, but **no reports of active surgical procedures for the region of the jaws.**[35] The assumption can be made that during his time the extraction of teeth was performed regularly. The following legend was written on a clay tablet by his court physician: *The inflammation wherewith his head, his hands and feet are inflamed is due to his teeth. His teeth must be extracted, it is on this account he is inflamed.*[36]

The earliest practice of the prosthetic arts was among the ancient Phoenicians circa 500 BC. Hammurapi, ruler of all lower Mesopotamia (1760 BC), established a state controlled economy in which fees charged by physicians were set. His law code contained two paragraphs dealing with teeth that show the high value placed on a tooth in those days:

"If a person knocks out the teeth of an equal, his teeth shall be knocked out."

"If he knocks out the tooth of a freed slave, he shall pay one third of a mine."[37] Teeth were knocked out as a form of punishment among these early people.

INDIA

The Brahmanic period marked the zenith of ancient Indian medicine. The earliest traces of medical writings are those of the so-called Bower manuscript, inscribed on birch bark approximately 400 AD which included 6 prescriptions for the care of the teeth and mouth.[38] Some of the diseases are ascribed etiologically to disproportions of the three fundamental humors (Dosha): Wind (Vayu), Bile (Pitta) and Mucus (Kapha, Shleshman) in accordance with the fundamentals of Indian Brahmanic medicine.[39]

All forms of gingival inflammation are described exactly by Sushruta. In the therapeutic part we find that they are cured with laxatives and emetics, scarification, application of herbal infusions and pastes with base of butter or honey.[40] Sushruta was keen on the

extraction of loose teeth only.[41] The removal of calculus **(sharkara)** was undertaken with a rhombus shaped instrument the periodontium being protected. Tooth extraction was done with a forceps called as **Samdamsha** or a kind of lever called as **Sharapunkhayantra**. There is no special description of fracture of the jaw. Luxations of the jaw are described in the section "Diseases of the teeth proper". The cause is "Wind", here elicited by loud speaking, chewing of hard substances and immoderate yawning.[42]

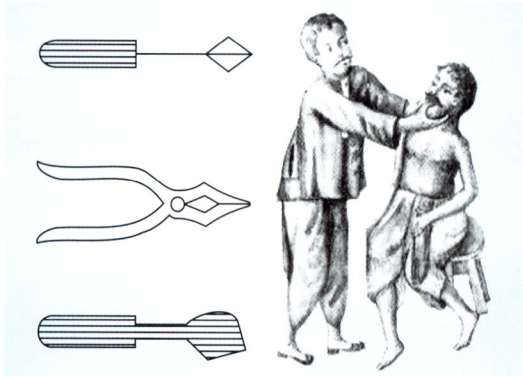

Fig. 2.4: Dental hygiene instrument **Dantalekhana/ Dantashanku** (left upper). Extraction forceps called as **Samdamsha** (left middle). Extraction instrument similar to lever called as **Sharapunkhayantra** (left lower). Procedure for mandibular reduction **Mukhopadhyaye** (right).

Not a single word was found in the Sanskrit literature about the replacement of extracted or crumbled teeth.[43]

THE GREEK AGE

Greek medicine was also a magic-religious-priest medicine in ancient times. True medicine started with the appearance of the **Father of medicine**. Hippocrates, who conducted a school for physicians where he taught rational medicine based on accumulated knowledge.[44] The contribution of the Greeks was mostly on the medical side. Because the Greek civilization was not a direct development of any preceding civilization, there was a smaller burden of magic to carry. The Greeks speculated on the operation of natural forces. They assumed that all life was derived from the real and natural base of nature.[45]

The ancient Greek physician, **Aesculapius**, who lived between 1300 and 1200 BC gained great frame for medical knowledge and skill. In time he was deified. Aesculapius originated the art of bandaging and use of purgatives. He also advocated cleaning of teeth and extractions. He is also credited with the concept of extracting diseased teeth.[46]

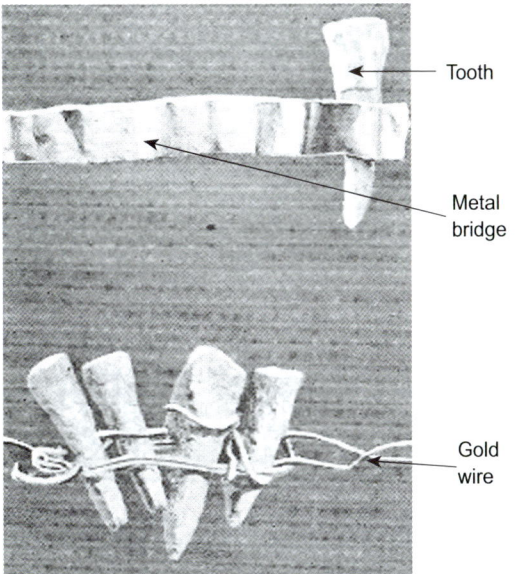

Fig. 2.5: Two **Greek appliances** existing in Archaeological museum of Athens.

Hippocrates (500 BC) was supposed to be a descendant of Aesculapius. Hippocrates became famous both as practitioner and writer on medical subjects. He did not believe in magic. He stressed nature's role in healing. Hippocrates raised the art of medicine to a high level. Also in one of his texts **(Peri-Arthron)** he devoted 32 paragraphs to the dentition. He appreciated the importance of teeth. He accurately described the technique for reducing a fracture of the jaw and also for replacing a dislocated mandible. He was familiar with extraction forceps for this is mentioned in one of his writings.[47] In his medical tomes he refers to accidents and illnesses affecting children during teething. Extraction of teeth is only recommended when teeth are actually loose: The principle of rational thought underlies the work of the Hippocratic school as is shown in the following case description: *When a person has an ulcer of long duration on the side of the tongue, one should examine the teeth on that side to see if one of them does not perhaps present a sharp point.* The ulcer is no longer simply accepted as a manifestation of divine displeasure, a logical cause is offered for its existence. In spite of the new logical approach to disease and the fact that organized magic was not practiced, old magic rites had not been abandoned completely. Medicinal preparations were not always of therapeutic value. The following grisly compound was recommended for halitosis in women: *Take the calcined head of a hare, three mice with their intestines removed but not the liver. Grind to a fine powder, mix with chalk and rub onto the teeth with unwashed wool. For toothache the bodies of mice were ground to a fine powder, mixed with marble and placed into the tooth cavity. Dog's teeth boiled in wine made a soothing mouthwash for a person suffering from tooth decay.* Unfortunately it has not been recorded whether these remedies actually alleviated suffering![48]

Aristotle (384–322 BC) followed Hippocrates. He was the representative of commonsense reasoning. He observed, classified his observations and sought out laws of nature. He accurately described extraction forceps and in his book **De Partibus Animal Culum** devoted a complete chapter to the teeth. He also stated figs and soft sweets produce decay. He called it a putrefactive process instead of fermentative.[49] Along with Hippocrates; he wrote of ointments and cautery with a red hot wire to treat diseases of the teeth and oral tissues (500–300 BC).[50] They advocated the use of wires to stabilize jaw fractures or to bind loose teeth. Although disproved, Aristotle's statement that men had more teeth than women, is surely one of the earliest recorded comparative dental anatomy observations. He further noted that the age of an animal could be determined by examining its teeth.[51]

The Greeks had a tooth numbering system that in principle corresponded to ours.[52] **MECHANICS** refers to the presence of a tooth forceps made of iron as an instrument of the physician known as ODONTAGRA. In addition the Greeks had **special root forceps** called as **RHIZAGRA**.[53]

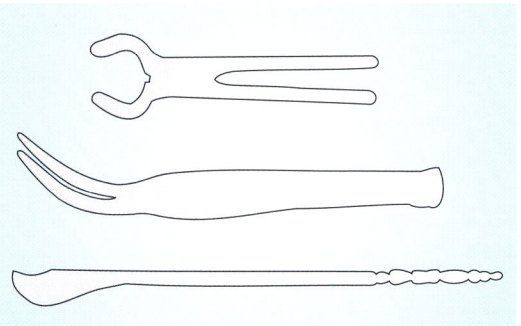

Fig. 2.6: Various ancient dental forceps and two other dental instruments existing in the Archaeological Museum of Athens.

equal of many made in Europe and America up until 1870 when the dental engine was invented. A very unusual specimen is a bridge constructed about 2500 years ago. This consists of several gold bands fastened to natural teeth and supporting three artificial teeth, two of which are made from a **calf's tooth** grooved in the center to appear like two central incisors. Etruscan art, seen at its best in Florence, reflects some oriental influence but essentially it is their own. Conquered in 309 BC, they were absorbed by the Roman Empire.[55]

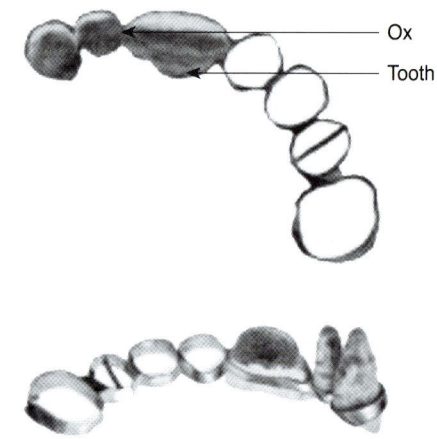

Ox

Tooth

Fig. 2.7: An **Etruscan appliance** for supporting three artificial teeth, two of which were made of one ox tooth, from front (above) and from back (below).

THE ETRUSCANS (100–400 BC)

Whereas the Greeks theorized on dental problems, the Etruscans were more practical and had skilled dentists. They were able to make dental appliances with exceptional skill. Partial dentures, of the bridgework type, were found in Etruscan tombs. Wide bands of pure gold were soldered together to fit over the natural teeth.[54] Etruscans, in the hills of Central Italy made the greatest contribution in restorative dentistry.

In Italian museums there are numerous specimens of crowns and bridges that were the

THE ROMAN AGE

The Romans absorbed the Etruscans and learnt their skills from them. They were not especially gifted in their dental art. They borrowed their medicine from the Greeks. Despite the advance in mechanical skill, superstition and magic had not yet been eradicated. Pliny the Elder's (23–79 AD). Natural History was the scientific textbook in use for many centuries. It contained many absurd remedies, e.g., a frog tied to the jaws would reputedly cause loose teeth to become firm again. One of his remedies for toothache, **plantago**, is still used today by homeopaths. Sporadic anatomical discoveries were made, viz Galen was the first person to speak of nerves in the teeth.[56]

Famous Roman physicians are named below:

Celsus (25 B C–50 AD) like Hippocrates did not believe in magic. He believed that General Physical deterioration caused dental diseases. For toothaches he prescribed hot water fomentations, narcotics, mustard seed, counter irritants, use of the cautery. He advocated the use of Alum for soft tissue disease and advised extraction of badly broken down teeth. He recommended filling the cavity with lead prior to extraction as a means of lessening the chance of fracturing the crown. He not only gave the technique for reduction of fractures but he was also the first to advocate the technique for tooth straightening or positioning. He also wrote extensively of oral diseases, including bleeding gums and ulcers of the oral cavity, as well as dental treatment such as narcotic-containing emollients and astringents.[57]

Archigenus (100 AD) recognized pulpitis and invented the dental drill to open into pulp chamber.[58]

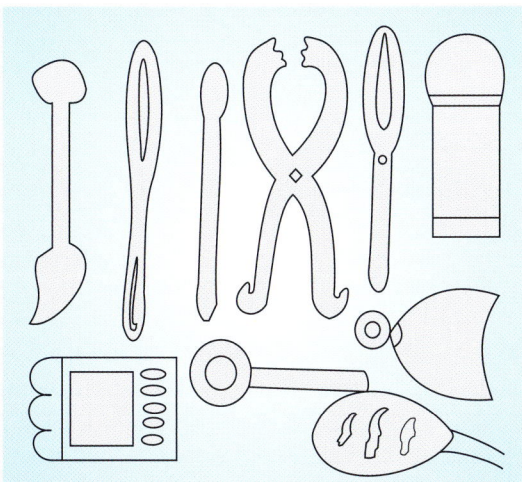

Fig. 2.8: Dental and surgical instruments represented in a funeral marble of the Lateran Museum, Rome.

Galen (200 A.D.) considered the greatest physician since Hippocrates, was the first to recognize that a toothache could be Pulpitis (inflammation of the pulp) or Pericementitis (inflammation of radicular portion of the tooth) He classified teeth into centrals, cuspids and molars.[59] He gave information on the use of bur to relieve tooth pain. He accurately described he insertion of the mandibular nerve in the mandibular canal through the foramen located near the molars, its course in the mandibular body and its exit on both sides of the symphysis.[60]

THE HEBREWS

As for the Hebrews, first evidence of dentistry among the Jews, relief of toothache and artificial restorations may be found in a collection of books known as **Talmud** (352 AD -407). In this collection, mention is made that women were more particular about facial appearance than were men. It stated that teeth were made of gold, silver and wood. The worm is blamed for decay. Also stated that gum disease started in the mouth but ended in the gut. One treatment for abscess was as follows:

Rx: Take earth near the outhouse, mix with honey then eat it.

As for extractions—all cultures expressed anxiety about removing a cuspid for fear of eye injury. This superstition continues today. The Hebrews are known for ethics, morals and religion. Despite numerous Hebrew writings that have survived, there is little written about dentistry.[61]

THE MIDDLE AGES

Arab civilization existed while Europe was in the Dark Ages; they reaped the fruits of contact between the secondary civilizations and were adept at the organization of this new knowledge. They soon established a cultured and wealthy Empire with centers of learning in places as far removed as Baghdad, Cairo and Cordova in Spain. Medical science was very highly developed; they were skilled in the use of anesthetics and applied some of the most difficult surgical procedures. Dentistry also benefited by this so-called organization of knowledge.[62]

Then came **Albucasis**, a Spanish moor of Cordova (1013 AD). He was considered the great exponent of dental surgery in the middle ages. He described extraction, scaling, reduction of fractures and the treatment of dislocated jaws in a treatise. In his book we find what was perhaps the first illustration of dental instruments. They were as follows:

1. 14 scalers
2. Elevators for surgery
3. Cautery
4. Forceps for surgery
5. Dental saws and files for removal of

caries. Besides being a famous surgeon and competent writer, he was also a greater teacher. He insisted on arriving at an accurate diagnosis. He believed in the referred pain theory. He accurately described technique for extractions, with special emphasis on careful manipulation of soft tissue. He also described treatment for partially luxated teeth. [63]

During the Islamic age, among the oral surgical procedures, the ranula operation is mentioned, being designated as frog under the tongue.[64]

Throughout the Middle Ages in Europe, dentistry was made available to wealthier individuals by physicians or surgeons who would go to the patient's home. Decay would sometimes be removed from teeth with a "dental drill," a metal rod that was rotated between the palms. Soft filling materials provided short-term alleviation of discomfort by keeping air from the open cavity. Dentistry for poorer people took place in the marketplace, where self-taught vagabonds would extract teeth for a small fee. From the Middle Ages to the early

1700s much dental therapy was provided by so called "barber surgeons." These jacks-of-all-trades would not only extract teeth and perform minor surgery, but they also cut hair, applied leeches to let blood, and performed embalming (treat to prevent it from decay).[65]

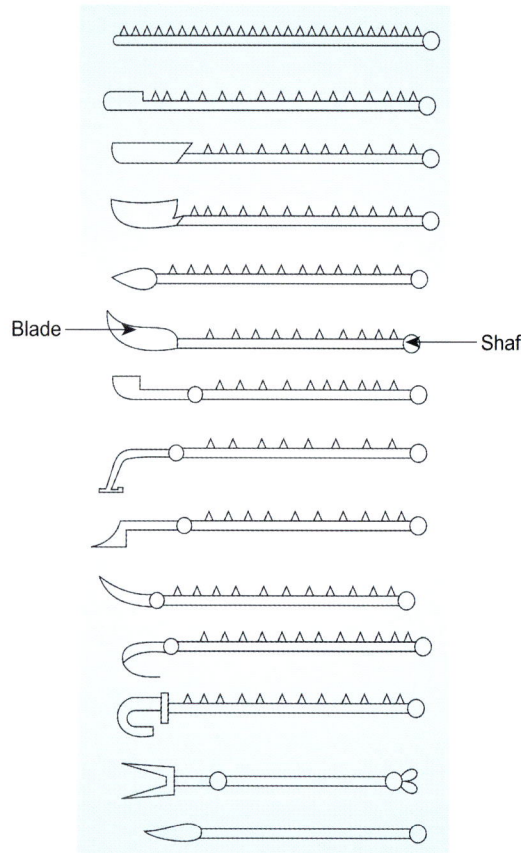

Fig. 2.9: The set of 14 **dental scrapers** of (Albucasis).

THE BARBER-SURGEONS

The Middle Ages witnessed the beginnings of the Guilds, among others the Guild of the Barber-Surgeons. In England where the craft of barber had been considered as honorable as that of surgeon, the Barber Surgeon's Guild was incorporated in the reign of Edward the Fourth. In 1540 this Guild joined that of the surgeons to become the United Company of Barber Surgeons, which existed as such until the mid-eighteenth century. Samuel Rutter was the last tooth drawer to be a master of the Barber-Surgeons.

In France the Barber-Surgeon's Guild dates from the 13th Century. It constituted the physicians, the grande bourgeoisie wearing square caps and long robes, haughtily pedantic. Of secondary importance were the petit bourgeoisie of clerical barber surgeons and finally the barbitonsores, a proletariat composed of lay barbers and outcast surgeons. In the Netherlands the position was much the same.

The question arises as to how the divergent activities of barber, surgeon and dentist were combined in the same guild. During the Middle Ages the influence and importance of the church cannot be underestimated. The artistic and cultural life was centered around the monasteries. The church spread its conception of labor and established order and method in work, which was given a certain dignity. Mediaeval Papal Edicts required monks and priests to be clean-shaven. Clerics were not allowed to perform bloody operations; consequently it became the duty of the layman barber, who was attached to the monastery, to officiate as the surgeon and dentist.[66]

Barbers had acted as assistants to the monks. When the pope in 1163 ruled that any operation involving the shedding of blood was incompatible with the priestly office, the barber took over the practice of Surgery. The barber surgeons were not the only ones doing extractions, another group made up of Vagabonds were known as **tooth drawers**. They plied their trade in public squares.[67] They often had very limited practical instruction and no scientific background at all. An isolated few of these barber surgeons held medical degrees. They wished to change the view that surgery and dentistry were handcrafts and therefore not suitable subjects to be taught at universities.

They wished to ally dentistry with surgery, and surgery with medicine. This eventually led to surgery becoming part of medicine, the surgeon being qualified in both fields. It follows that in Western Europe, dentistry as a part of surgery, could only be practiced by people with a medical qualification. Doctores Medicinae were trained at universities; a person therefore legally qualified to practice dentistry was a fully qualified medical doctor and surgeon. A person so qualified, would not be likely to confine himself exclusively to dentistry, then considered a subsidiary subject.

The emergent science suffered a setback, as the field was now wide open for charlatans and quacks. While the barber-surgeon operated in the urban areas, the trades of barber and bloodletter were left to the blacksmith and shoemaker in the country districts. They handled the extractions, assisted by itinerant toothdrawers who visited the market places from time to time. Drums were played loudly to drown the shrieks of the victims, which could frighten prospective patients away. The itinerant tooth drawer eventually disappeared from the village scene and is today only to be found in isolated places like Morocco, plying his trade on the busy Market Square. Guy de Chauliac (1309–1368), himself a barber-surgeon, wrote in his book **Chirurgia Magna** that barbers and dentatores were operating on the teeth and doing extractions. Two centuries later Herman Ryff of Strasbourg wrote a monograph in which dental afflictions were dealt with under a separate heading.[68]

THE RENAISSANCE PERIOD (14TH–16TH CENTURY)

The Renaissance brought a general revival in learning; dentistry shared in the intellectual awakening. As in all scientific fields, an effort was made to shake off ancient and mediaeval magic rites, superstitions and unscientific beliefs. The economic revolution had brought the means to enable certain men to devote their time and energies to study and experimenting. Science began to influence their mental processes. Acute observation led them to abandon abstract myths. Textbooks written during the 16th and 17th centuries became more practical.

Ambrose Pare, known as the **father of modern surgery,** was a barber's apprentice. He was surgeon to Henry II, Frances II and Charles IX as well as Henry III. He wrote prolifically and was the author of an illustrated practical treatise on dentistry. It is significant that this treatise was written by the surgeon to the French Court. Dentistry was therefore still firmly under the wing of surgery. Pare's realistic description of extractions was not very encouraging to would be patients. The first textbook to be published in English was written by **Charles Allen** in 1685, viz. **The Operator for the Teeth.**[69]

Around 1300 universities like those at Paris, Oxford and Bologna were founded and

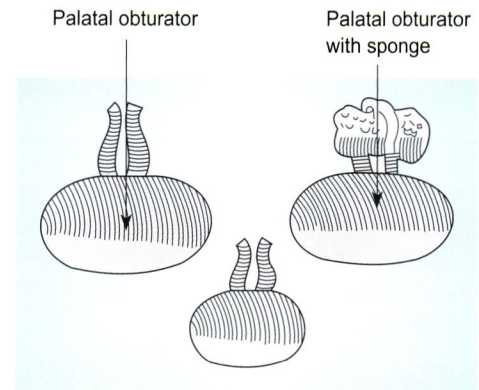

Fig. 2.11: The **palatine obturator with sponge** of Ambrose Pare.

important books made their appearance. In **Chirurgia Magna**, the French surgeon **Guy de Chauliac** devoted some space to pathology and therapeutics of the teeth. Chauliac was first to coin the term dentator and dentists. The English term dentist came from his original terms. Following Chauliac came **Giovanni de Arcoli** in 1400. His opinions and instruments were somewhat modern. His **pelican** for extraction of teeth was used for years and his root forceps could be used today. He advised good oral cleaning habits and to avoid hot and cold substances and sweet **stuffs**. He was first to mention filling teeth with gold.

Most of the great surgeons had no knowledge of Anatomy but their teachings were not refuted until **Vesalius**, 1500 of Belgium, rebelled and became an anatomist at the University of Padua, Italy. He freed the mind of the medical profession and laid the foundation for true scientific research, which is the basis of our present day medical practice. He accurately described the teeth and pulp chambers. **Fallopius** was another anatomist, a pupil of Vesalius. He is credited with the descriptions of the dental follicle, trigeminal nerve, auditory nerve, LX nerve, the glossopharyngeal, and hard and soft palate. He stated that teeth were not true bone.

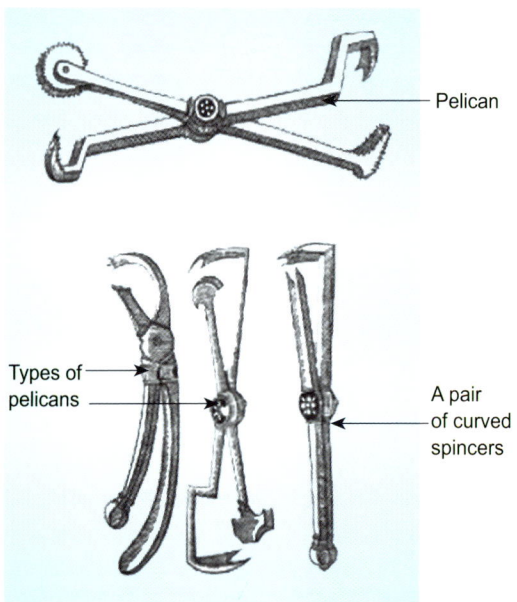

Fig. 2.10: The various **pelicans** used by Ambrose Pare.

Eustachius (1500) gave a complete anatomical description of teeth and their development, the periodontal membrane and alveoli. He was credited with the first complete dental book, ninety-five pages of anatomy, embryology, physiology, blood and nerve supply of the teeth. In this text, he completely describes the anatomy of the teeth, their development, the alveolus and the periodontal membrane.

Leonardo da Vinci (end of 15th Century) described the anatomy of the jaws, teeth and maxillary sinus. These drawings are the first to accurately describe the maxillary sinus. However, credit has been given to **Dr. Nathaniel Highmore** of England (1650).

Ambroise Pare (16th Century) was born in Paris. He was a barber-surgeon at 16 years of age and became a member of the College of Surgeons at age 37. He was the first to describe palatal obturators, and transplant techniques, etc. His instruments though crude could be used today. He was not interested in restorative dentistry. He believed toothache was due to worms attacking the teeth.[70]

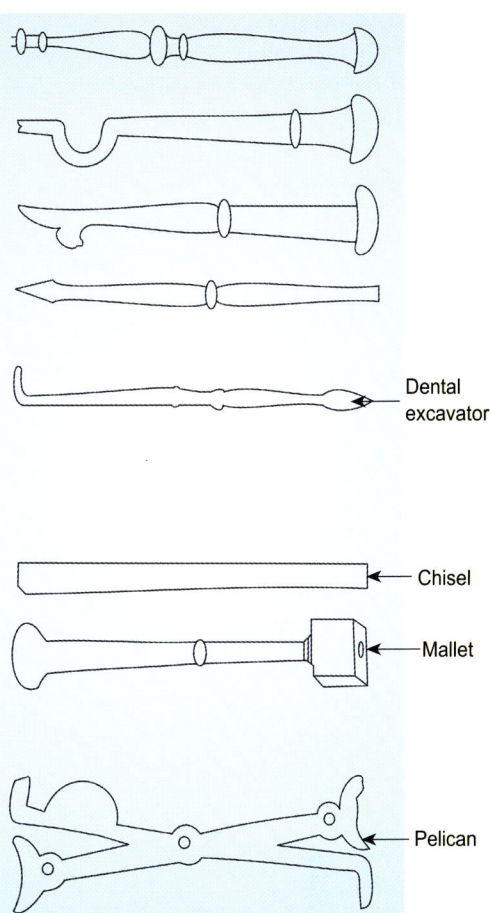

Dental excavator

Chisel

Mallet

Pelican

Fig. 2.13: Instruments used in modern times showing a *pelican* (last instrument) a *chisel and a mallet* (2nd and 3rd instrument from below) used in those times for the extraction of tooth.

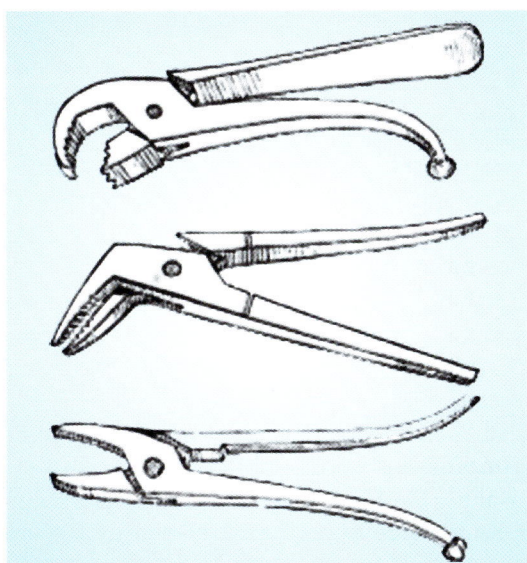

Fig. 2.12: Different kinds of forceps used in the 16th century

SEVENTEENTH CENTURY

Leeuwenhoek (17th Century) invented the microscope. He described the dental tubuli and was the first to see organisms of the mouth. **Malpighi** (17th Century) a great Italian anatomist was founder of histology and made great use of the microscope for tissue studies. F.M. Bourdet (mid 18th Century) described use of gold for baseplates.

Purman of Breslau (middle 17th Century) is known for wax impressions.

Charles Goodyear (1840) discovered vulcanite rubber. It was used for denture bases. This discovery led to false teeth for the millions. Dentures were called vulcanite dentures. **Philip Pfaff** (18th Century) a German introduced plaster for pouring up models

J.E.J. Dunning (1844) is credited with plaster of Paris impressions, first shown in America. **John Greenwood** (1789) made dentures for George Washington.[71]

EIGHTEENTH CENTURY

During the l8th Century France led the dental field and **Pierre Fauchard** was given the retrospective title **The Father of Scientific Dentistry** for his comprehensive work **Le Chirurgien Dentiste**, which covered almost everything connected with the subject of dentistry in the l8th Century. He wrote that most celebrated surgeons did not wish to practice dentistry. The technical training required to fill and replace teeth was not to their

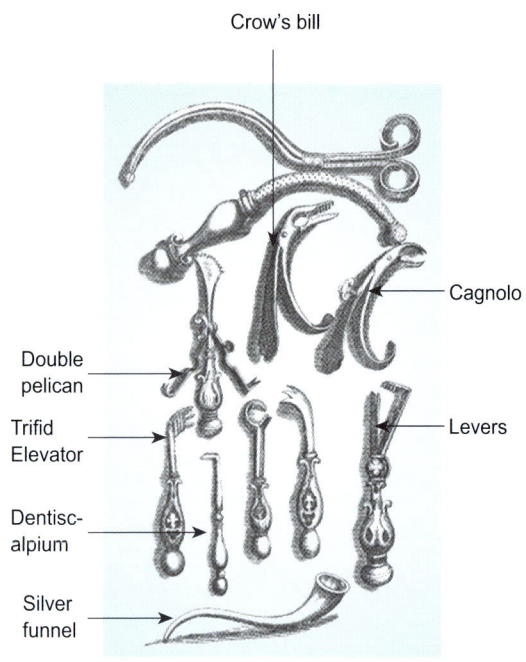

Crow's bill

Cagnolo

Double pelican

Trifid Elevator

Levers

Dentisc-alpium

Silver funnel

Fig. 2.14: Several dental instruments used in the 17th century.

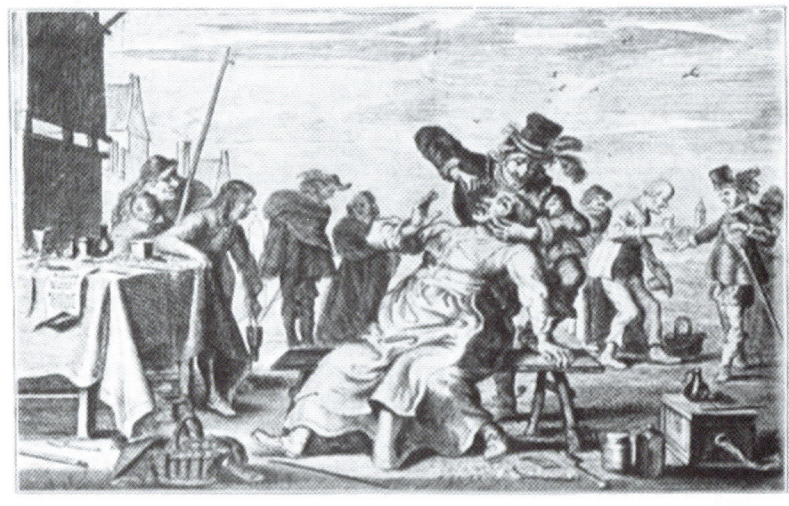

Fig. 2.15: Tooth drawer at a public place in Holland.

taste. This was unfortunately to the detriment of the public as untrained people now turned to dentistry.[72]

He also wrote a complete work on Odontology in two volumes, 843 pages. He recognized the intimate relationship between oral conditions and general health. He advocated the use of lead (plombagel) to fill cavities. He removed all decay and if the pulp was exposed, he used the cautery. He prescribed oil of cloves and cinnamon for pulpitis. He described partial dentures and full dentures in his text. He constructed dentures with springs and used human teeth. Gold dowels were used in root canals filled with lead. He was also known as **Father of Orthodontics**. Fauchard died in 1768 at the age of 83.[73]

Following Fauchard's work Robert **Bunon** (1743) printed the first dental therapeutics text, dentistry's first pharmacopoeia. **John Hunter** authored "Natural History of the Human Teeth" in 1771. **Thomas Berdmore** was credited with "Disorders and Deformities of Teeth and Gums" in 1768. **Joseph Fox**—Pupil of Hunter; wrote text, same title "Natural History of the Human Teeth". He amplified the work of his teacher and influenced dentistry in England and U.S. These men on the continent and in England were not physicians or surgeons writing on the teeth but dentists recording their observations.[74]

The profession of dentistry suffered a severe setback during the French Revolution. The Republic was declared in September 1793, followed by the Reign of Terror with the Committee of Public Safety as its instrument. Complete control was exercised over the external and internal affairs of France. The Jacobeans reorganized France. Much was retrograde and oppressive, for example, all control was removed from the practice of the professions, namely medicine, surgery, law and emergent dentistry. In 1792 the universities, faculties and learned societies were suppressed, consequently any person could now practice these professions. Chaos ensued until the problem was solved by Napoleon Bonaparte in 1802, when he made all such practitioners officers of state. Dentistry was officially classified as a speciality of surgery and for 100 years the dental profession in France possessed no charter. Two dental schools were established in 1880 and 1884. Meanwhile, the New World was being colonized. It has been established that by 1736 dental training was included in the curriculum of the French Naval School at Rocheport. The naval surgeons trained at these and other similar naval schools had to serve in the colonies for three years. They were only taught to extract teeth. According to Weinburger, Le Mayeur (Lemair) of the French forces introduced the dentistry of Pierre Fauchard to America.[75]

NINETEENTH CENTURY

Poor communications made instruction in the craft very difficult, itinerant dentists could not pass on their knowledge to anybody else. This was the position in 1830. In 1839 the Baltimore College of Dental Surgery was founded by two American dentists, Horace H. Hayden (1769-1844) and Chapin. A. Harris. The standard of dentistry was gradually improved by raising the standard of the curriculum and exams. John Harris of Bainbridge, Ohio, was the founder of the Ohio College of Dental Surgery in Cincinnati. The Universities would not integrate the dental schools with their medical faculties, with the result that many dental schools in America became private ventures. **The American Journal of Dental Science** was published in **1839** in Baltimore on the instigation of Eleazer Parmly of New York and Chapin A. Harris of Baltimore. The University of Maryland recognized the **DDS** degree and the precedent were established that a dentist could use the title Doctor. This was to have repercussions in South Africa in the 20th century. In 1840 the first **American Society of Dental Surgeons** was started in New York with Horace H. Hayden as the first president.

Warner comments that by the mid-nineteenth century, dentistry in America was synonymous with the turnkey. This can best be described as a primitive tool like a ratchet wrench used for extracting teeth. With improved communications and the new dental schools, the position changed for the better, with the result that many Europeans made use of the improved facilities in America. There were so many American dentists practicing in Europe that leading figures met in Switzerland in 1873 to establish **The American Dental Society of Europe** for dentists legally qualified in America. This society paved the way for the **Federation Dentaire International** which did much to facilitate the progress of the profession. The members of the newly formed "American Dental Society of Europe" wished to stop unqualified persons from advertising their practices as "American Dental Institutions".

In England **John Hunter's** contribution to dental literature **The Natural History of Human Teeth** (1771) is interesting from the point of view that various methods of transplanting human teeth are described in great detail. Hunter is referred to by Rowlett as a pathologist and surgeon, and by Woodforde as a brilliant general surgeon and anatomist. Although there is some doubt as to his exact profession, this "key figure" **was no dentist.** In 1858 legislation clarified the position somewhat. The Medical Act of that year made it legal for the Queen to grant a charter to the Royal College of Surgeons to award licenses in dentistry. In 1878 the first Dentist's Act provided for a register to be kept by the General Medical Council. The Odontological Society was formed in Britain with the British Journal of Dental Science as its organ. In the late l9th century (1880-1890) the dentist was rated low on the social scale in most centers. Ennis particularly blames the activities of unethical American dentists on the continent for this situation.[76]

REFERENCES AND BIBLIOGRAPHY

19. History of Dentistry 2001 by Terry Wilwerdin 3.
20. *Idem.*
21. *Idem.*
22. History of Dentistry 2001 by Terry Wilwerding 4.
23. The History of Dentistry in South Africa 1652-1900 by Dr Vilma Grobler 1.
24. *Idem.*
25. History of Dentistry by Walter Hoffman-Axthelm, 1981,Chapter 1, 19.
26. The History of Dentistry in South Africa 1652–1900 by Dr Vilma Grobler 3.
27. History of Dentistry by Walter Hoffman-Axthelm, 1981, Chapter 1, 23.
28. History of Dentistry 2001 by Terry Wilwerding 4.
29. History of Dentistry by Walter Hoffman-Axthelm, 1981, Chapter 1, 22.
30. History of Dentistry by Walter Hoffman-Axthelm, 1981, Chapter 1, 24.
31. History of Dentistry by Walter Hoffman-Axthelm, 1981, Chapter 1, 26.
32. History of Dentistry by Walter Hoffman-Axthelm, 1981, Chapter 3, 42.
33. History of Dentistry 2001 by Terry Wilwerding 4.
34. History of Dentistry by Walter Hoffman-Axthelm, 1981, Chapter 3, 43.
35. History of Dentistry by Walter Hoffman-Axthelm, 1981, Chapter 1, 27.
36. The History of Dentistry in South Africa 1652–1900 by Dr Vilma Grobler 3.
37. History of Dentistry 2001 by Terry Wilwerding 4.
38. History of Dentistry by Walter Hoffman-Axthelm, 1981, Chapter 2, 36.
39. History of Dentistry by Walter Hoffman-Axthelm, 1981, Chapter 2, 37.
40. *Idem.*
41. History of Dentistry by Walter Hoffman-Axthelm, 1981, Chapter 2, 38.
42. History of Dentistry by Walter Hoffman-Axthelm, 1981, Chapter 2, 39.
43. History of Dentistry by Walter Hoffman-Axthelm, 1981, Chapter 2, 40.
44. History of Dentistry by Walter Hoffman-Axthelm, 1981, Chapter 5, 60.
45. The History of Dentistry in South Africa 1652–1900 by Dr Vilma Grobler 3.

46. History of Dentistry 2001 by Terry Wilwerding 4.
47. *Idem.*
48. The History of Dentistry in South Africa 1652–1900 by Dr Vilma Grobler 4.
49. History of Dentistry 2001 by Terry Wilwerding 4.
50. The History of Dentistry in South Africa 1652–1900 by Dr Vilma Grobler 1.
51. Idem.
52. History of Dentistry by Walter Hoffman-Axthelm, 1981, Chapter 5, 61.
53. History of Dentistry by Walter Hoffman-Axthelm, 1981, Chapter 5, 65, 66.
54. The History of Dentistry in South Africa 1652–1900 by Dr Vilma Grobler 4
55. History of Dentistry 2001 by Terry Wilwerding 5
56. The History of Dentistry in South Africa 1652–1900 by Dr Vilma Grobler 5.
57. History of Dentistry 2001 by Terry Wilwerding 5.
58. *Idem.*
59. *Idem.*
60. History of Dentistry by Walter Hoffman-Axthelm, 1981, Chapter 5, 74, 75.
61. History of Dentistry 2001 by Terry Wilwerding 5.
62. The History of Dentistry in South Africa 1652–1900 by Dr Vilma Grobler 6.
63. History of Dentistry 2001 by Terry Wilwerding 6.
64. History of Dentistry by Walter Hoffman-Axthelm, 1981, Chapter 7, 100.
65. The History of Dentistry in South Africa 1652-1900 by Dr Vilma Grobler 1.
66. The History of Dentistry in South Africa 1652-1900 by Dr Vilma Grobler 7.
67. History of Dentistry 2001 by Terry Wilwerding 6.
68. The History of Dentistry in South Africa 1652–1900 by Dr Vilma Grobler 8.
69. *Idem.*
70. History of Dentistry 2001 by Terry Wilwerding 6.
71. History of Dentistry 2001 by Terry Wilwerding 7.
72. The History of Dentistry in South Africa 1652–1900 by Dr Vilma Grobler 11.
73. History of Dentistry 2001 by Terry Wilwerding 7.
74. *Idem.*
75. The History of Dentistry in South Africa 1652–1900 by Dr Vilma Grobler 11.
76. The History of Dentistry in South Africa 1652–1900 by Dr Vilma Grobler 11.

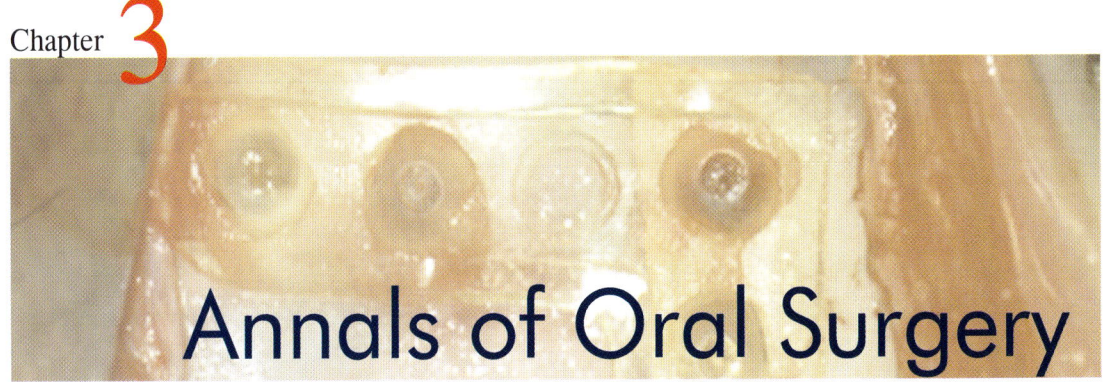

Chapter 3

Annals of Oral Surgery

Oral surgery is just one part of the whole field of dentistry. It deals with such a diversity of conditions and procedures and covers such a vast area of study that it has by necessity become an area of specialization.

A BRIEF HISTORY OF ORAL SURGERY

Oral surgery begins with the Egyptians in about 1600 BC and was later refined by the Greeks who brought a scientific approach to medicine in around 500 BC. They even developed a type of dental forceps. The Romans contributed to the area and then it wasn't until the 1500's in France where we find French surgeon Ambroise Paré who described a method of transplanting and re-implanting teeth. He also developed methods of handling cleft or perforated palates, extracting teeth, draining abscesses and setting jaw fractures.

Oral surgery began serious and more structured development in America in the 19th and 20th centuries. This was a period where a variety of guilds, societies and groups in specialized fields were trying to grasp complete control to direct and license their members. Printers, masons, shipwrights and carpenters were no different than the professional associations in the medical and dental fields.

The American Medical Association determined that Oral Surgeons could only be doctors and not dentists. They demanded that only someone holding an MD degree could be a surgeon. As time went on there was a gradual acceptance that a dentist must not necessarily hold an MD degree in order to practice Oral Surgery.

The Civil War, World War I and World War II provided arenas where dentists were required to not only remove or repair teeth but to assist in and conduct surgical procedures in areas dealing with the jaw, mouth and faces of victims of battle. They, closed wounds, applied anesthetics and helped in the sorting of casualties.

Following World War I the Society of Oral and Cosmetic Surgeons was formed although it largely consisted of doctors holding dual degrees in medicine and dentistry. World War II saw the formation of maxillofacial surgical teams to deal with injuries to the faces and jaws of soldiers.

Each team was to consist of an oral surgeon, a plastic surgeon, a surgical nurse, an anesthetist and supporting personnel. A lack of plastic surgeons required oral surgeons to provide complete care, including cosmetic surgery that was intended for the soldiers. They met with remarkable success.

Following the war the American Medical Association again pushed for control of oral surgery training and licensing. The American Board of Oral Surgery had been formed in 1946 and they established standards that could only be met in hospital residency programs.

The Army and Air Force gradually built and established their own oral surgery residency programs with the cooperation of medical and dental schools. Through time the standards for oral surgeons has increased to its present state of excellence.

Oral surgeons are possibly the best-trained and most knowledgeable practitioners when it comes to the face, jaw and neck. They have been doing reconstructive surgery, plastic surgery and oral surgery in some form or other since the First World War, intensely during the Second World War and their training and residency programs are at a recognized state of excellence.

EVOLUTION OF TECHNIQUES IN ORAL SURGERY

Tooth Extraction

The earliest mention in our cultural sphere of the extraction of a tooth, offering relief from toothache with relative certainty of success, is surprisingly found only in the Hippocratic writings, and is followed with a minute description by the Roman Celsus in the first century AD. Two centuries later Galen recommended medicamentous preparation-loosening the tooth with etching agents, a method which was given preference more and more with the hemophobic Islamic physicians. Albucasis alone represented an exception to this. This etching therapy was adopted by the majority of physicians and surgeons in the Middle Ages. When any of them described the surgical extraction, however, from Guy de Chauliac, who was the first to mention the pelican, to Ambroise Pare, he adhered to the procedure described by Abulcasim. The actual performance of the procedure, however, until far into modern times remained in the hands of the tooth-drawers and lower barber-surgeons. In the 18th century, Fauchard gave a precise description of instruments used for extracting teeth and the books of Jourdain, also in France, and of Bucking in Germany concerned themselves especially with dental surgery.

The 19th century had its beginning in this subject with the book, "Des accidents de l'extraction des dents" (Accidents in the Extraction of Teeth), published in 1802 by the Maitre en Chirurgie and dentist Jacques Rene Duval, the biographer of Jourdain and author of a history of dentistry. Endowed with a rich knowledge of literature, extending from Hippocrates to his own contemporaries, he described all possible complications in 93 well-organized pages. He arrived at the conclusion that accidents were not usually the fault of the well-trained dentist, but rather the result of external circumstances. Therefore the dentist need not have too great a fear of this procedure.

The preferred instruments of the first half of the century were pelicans, levers, keys, dental forceps, and curved-shank elevators, the first three of which extensively traumatized the tissue surrounding the tooth. In order to eliminate this disadvantage, as already mentioned, almost all authors especially strove to improve the pelican. This instrument was so popular in Germany that in 1781 it served the former regimental medical officer Friedrich Schiller as a metaphor in his play "Die Rauber" (The Robbers). Mention of it is lacking, however, in the English language literature of the 19th century:

Joseph Fox in 1806 limited himself essentially to the key, and Thomas Bell in 1826 restricted himself to the key, the forceps, and the lever. Fox spoke of the "German key", while the surgeon Benjamin Bell claimed the instrument for his own country. Regarding the nomenclature of this key we have been informed by the discussion of Johann Jacob Joseph Serre. Added to this was the pyramid-shaped root screw, also first described by Serre in 1803, and named after him. It is a matter of a dozen threaded screws which, depending on size, are screwed into the remainder of the root. Then, after a handle had

been screwed on, it was pulled out much like a corkscrew. The idea of this root-screw was passed along chiefly by Simon P. Hullihen in West Virginia in 1844.

He was **the first important** oral surgeon in the modern sense. For the removal of the roots of maxillary anterior teeth, he combined a screw with a compound root forceps to avoid collapse

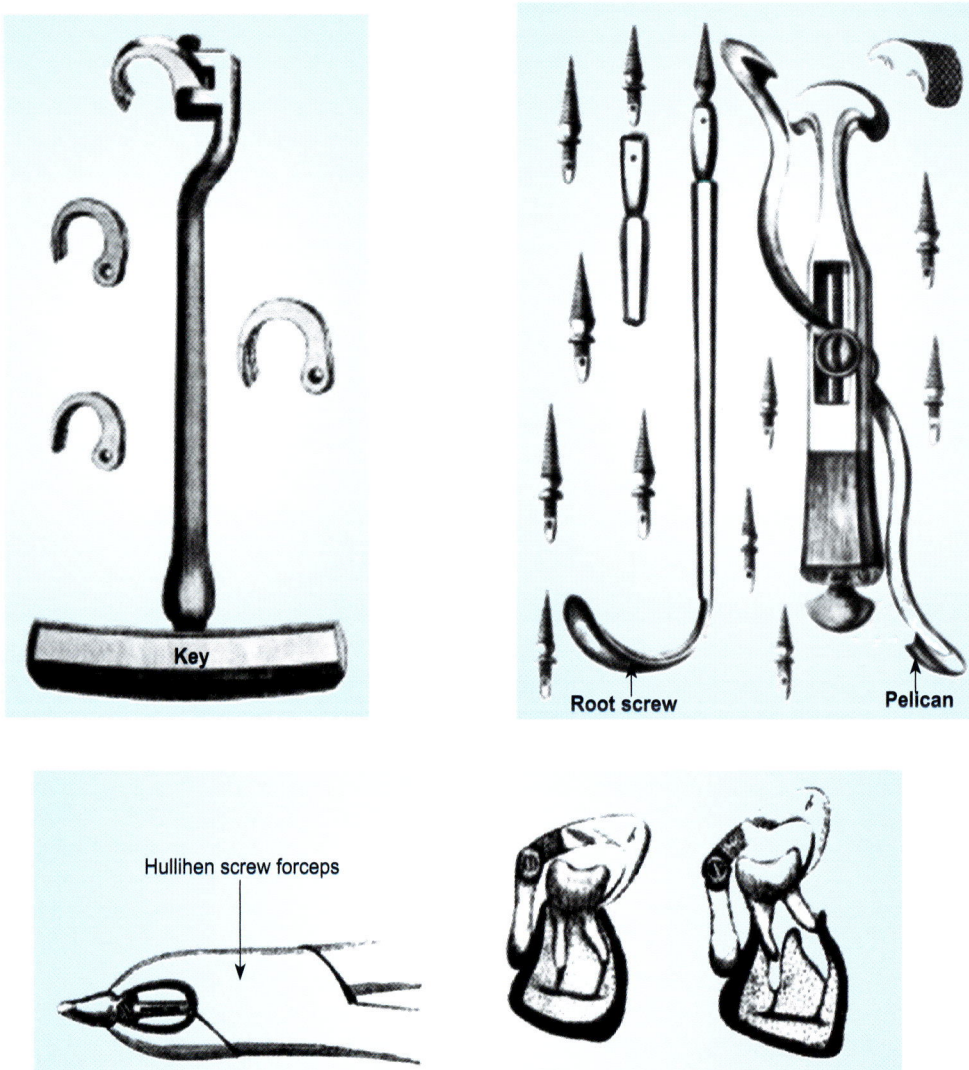

Fig. 3.1: Laforgue key, *1802* (upper left) **Serre's root screw and pelican,** 1803 (upper right) mode of action of key, 1815 (lower right) and **Hullihen screw forceps** for root extraction, 1844 (lower left)

of the root under the pressure of the forceps. A combination between forceps and key was mentioned in an essay published in London in 1826 and in Leipzig in 1827 by de la Fons, a dentist active in London. In 1836 the Berlin dentist Eduard Blume pronounced the lever as antiquated and the pelican as indispensable. Even in 1843 Desirabode in Paris called the key (clef de Garengeot) the most widely used instrument, which he, however, had personally done without for a long time. The forceps (pince), straight or curved, is used essentially for the anterior teeth, the crow's bill (davier) for the molars, the goat's foot elevator (pied-de-biche) for the roots, and the lever of Lecluse (langue-de-carpe) for the third molars, in all cases in both maxilla and mandible.

Desirabode believed that the pelican was no longer in general use except by a few practitioners and in northern Europe. In the forties of this century dental surgery received new impulses on one hand through the introduction of anesthesia and on the other through the development of anatomically shaped forceps by John Tomes in London. If we examine, for example, the forceps of Louis Laforgue of Paris from 1802, we see that this type of instrument had undergone few changes since the days of Ambroise Pare, some 250 years before. In the June, 1841 issue of the London Medical Gazette Tomes published a paper on the correct construction and use of forceps. At first the contemporary set of instruments is described. As with Thomas Bell, the forceps are for the anterior teeth, the key is for the molars, and the elevator if all else fails. It is to be noted that Tomes decisively rejects the key. Especially, however, he finds the forceps insufficient. They should grip the tooth only, and the force should be brought to bear in the axis of the tooth.

For each group of teeth, therefore, a forceps must be available which corresponds to their anatomical shape. Forceps should be constructed and used upon the principle of lengthening the tooth for the extraction of which they are intended; thus enabling the operator to move it from side to side, or rotate it if the fang be single, and of a shape admitting of such motion. After these lateral movements have been produced the tooth may, unless the fangs have some peculiar position or shape, be raised in a perpendicular direction, leaving as little injury from its removal as the operation can admit. According to his own principles Tomes constructed a set of anatomically shaped forceps, and therewith elevated this device, which had been neglected up to that point, to dentistry's most important extraction instrument today.

It was an especially fortunate circumstance that he found a superb instrument maker in Jean-Marie Evrard, born in Toulouse and a former student of the famous Charriere in Paris who had been working in London since 1837. For the removal of roots Tomes later recommended the straight and curved levers in his textbook of 1859. Tomes' forceps shapes retained their validity for the entire century. Recommended improvements, such as the bent-down handle, found no lasting acceptance. After an even closer physical contact of the gripping devices on the cervix of the tooth was achieved (Berten 1905), the dental forceps had reached the form in which they have been used ever since.

Oral Surgery

The field of clinical oral surgery, which is so extensive today, was founded in the forties of the last century by Simon P.Hullihen, who established the first specialized clinic for the field in Wheeling, West Virginia. According to his notes he had operated about 150 hare-lips and cleft palates, 150 cancers, 200 antrum cases, 25 cases of making new noses, 50 new lips, and 10 underjaws, but also 300 cases of cataract and strabismus and 200 cases of general surgery. Well known is his report on the surgical elimination

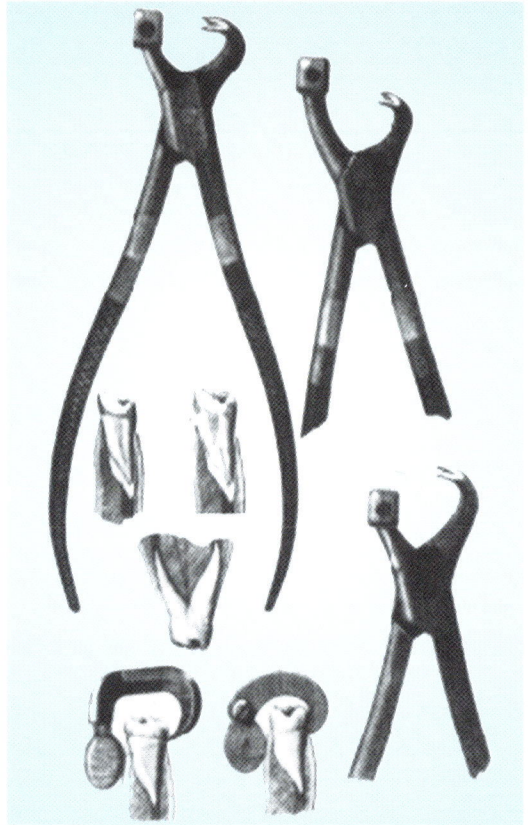 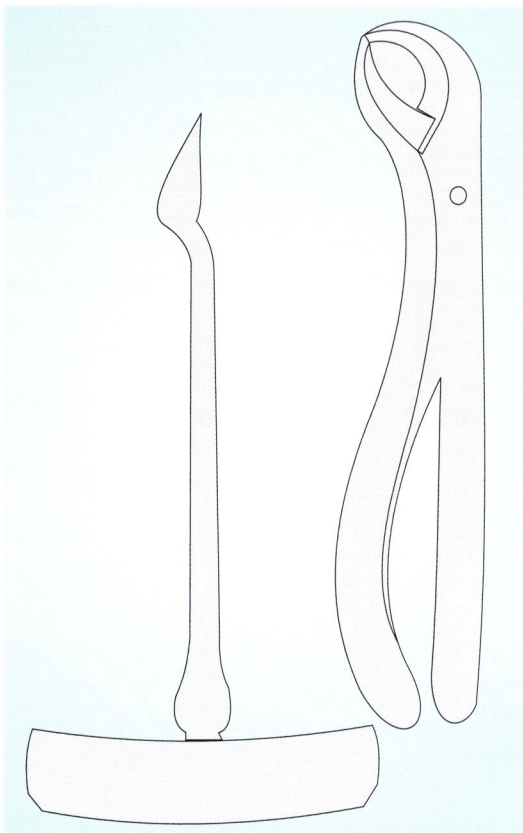

Fig. 3.2: A combination of **forceps and key,** 1825 **(De La Fons)** (left) **La Forgue elevator** *(from Lecluse) and* **forceps,**1802 (right)

of an alveolar protrusion of the mandible through mobilization and repositioning of the anterior part of the alveolar process including the teeth, and all this alone in the last ten years of his short life. On methodology he reported in dental journals.

James Edward Garretson, who practiced in Philadelphia and whose clinic was associated with the Dental College there, soon followed Hullihen's path. Through his success in operations, but mainly through his work **A Treatise on the Diseases and Surgery of the Mouth, Jaws and Associate Parts**, which was published in 1869 and which underwent six editions through 1895 under the title **A System of Oral Surgery**, he established jaw

surgery as an independent field. It was proved very quickly that men such as Hullihen and Garretson, who were skillful dentists and physicians, had obtained operative results completely different from those of the general surgeons. Their familiarity with intraoral work and their knowledge of dental technique made it possible for them to construct the auxiliary apparatuses necessary for surgical procedures on the jaw.

Within the scope of this book, we can only concern ourselves with the systematic development of specialized outpatient dental surgery. Besides local anesthesia, which was coming gradually into general use in the nineties, the discovery by Wilhelm Conrad

Roentgen in Wurzburg of the phenomenon of X-rays on November 8, 1895, was of decisive importance. The first photographs of teeth were made already on the 2nd of February 1896 by the Frankfurt physicist WalterKonig and also, probably only a few days later, with the help of a physicist there, Friedrich Giesel, by Otto Walkhoff, a dentist then still practicing in Braunschweig. The first radiographs of teeth in the United States followed one year after Roentgen's discovery by the dentist C. Edmund Kells, who became one of the many martyrs to this diagnostic aid. Because of an X-ray cancer originating from his fingers and continually recurring, he parted from life. He shot himself.

What had been achieved previously in dental surgery were acts of individual virtuosity by surgically talented dentists more than therapeutic methods of general importance. Nevertheless, these pioneer deeds ought not to be underrated because they formed the basis for dentistry to develop from the exclusively practiced tooth extraction to a standard far beyond the limits of thousands of years.

The first description of a procedure called the "apicectomy" in English, "Wurzelspitzen-resektion" in German, and in French "resection apicale" belongs to this development. We find an early mention of it in a report from 1880 on a lecture given by John Nutting Farrar in New York. Four years earlier he had recommended treating chronic processes at the apex by means of injections through it. He still advised this method for the anterior teeth or if a fistula was present, but for the inaccessible molars he recommended penetrating with a drill from the oral vestibule to the apical site of inflammation to create an artificial fistula, a method which, although seldom used today, is called "apicotomy".

Then, in 1884, Farrar published on the basis of nine years of experience his radical and heroic method of amputating more or less large parts of the root or even of the whole root of a molar with simultaneous filling of the root canal. At about the same time similar suggestions were made by Charles William Dunn, Claude Martin, and chiefly by Meyer Louis Rhein in New York in 1890.

The credit for the methodical development of apicectomy under cocaine anesthesia in the years 1895 to 1899 belongs to the professor of the University of Breslau, Carl Partsch, a surgeon who had turned to dentistry. The Viennese professor Rudolf Weiser joined him and propagated Partsch's method at the IIIrd International Dental Congress in Paris in 1900. At about the same time Partsch introduced the curved incision named after him, which is still predominantly used today. It was not until 1908, however, that he recommended closing the wound with silk thread.

Partsch also earned particular credit in the field of cyst operations. We remember the treatment of Scultetus, Fauchard, Runge, and Jourdain of such hollow tumors, which they took mostly for an abscess. In 1829 a report from the surgical clinic at the Hotel Dieu in Paris, then under the direction of Guillaume Dupuytren, mentioned bone cysts (kystes osseux) in the jaw region as if it was a matter of course in discussing a case from 20 years before. Through pressure on the tumor, Dupuytren produced a light crepitation, a feeling similar to that of paper rumpled between the fingers, or, even better, very dry parchment, (which is), according to M. Dupuytren, the pathognomonic indication for this affliction. This symptom still bears the name today of this great surgeon, who was one of the first who dared to perform a mandibular resection. As further diagnostic aid the exploratory puncture was used. The therapy consisted in a wide opening and removal of the edges of the bone, irrigation with etching substances and packing in order to destroy the membrane of the sinus by infection. In the case of recurrences he employed the cautery to pull up everything by the roots.

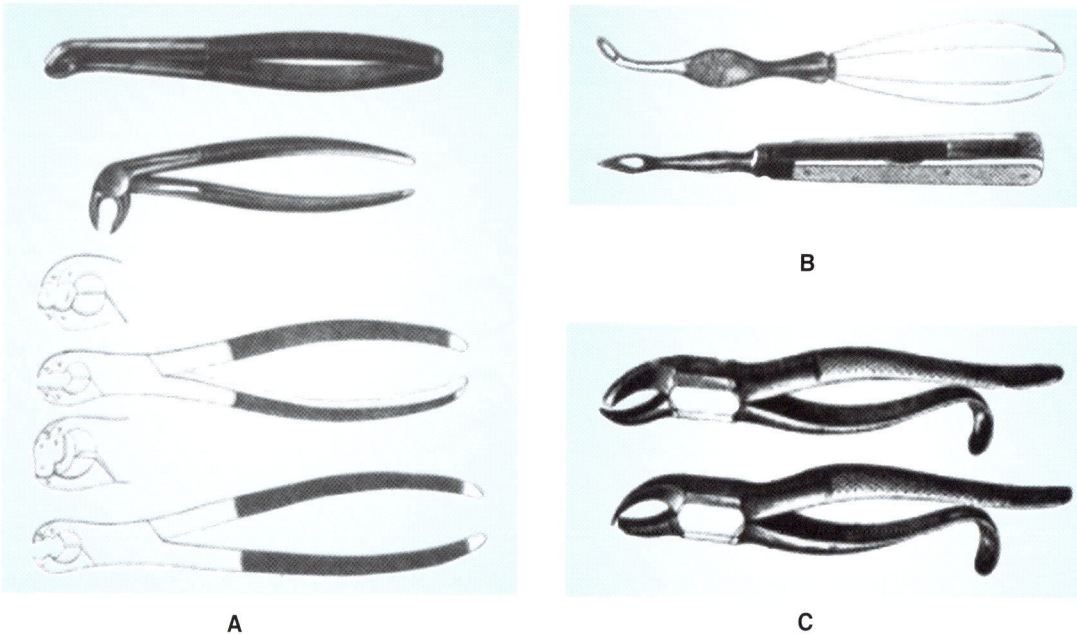

Fig. 3.3: (A) Sketches and finished designs of **Tomes' forceps,** 1841; (B) **Tomes' elevator,** 1859; (C) **Forceps handles of Read** (Ash Catalogue, 1898)

In 1892 Partsch recommended that cysts lined with epithelium be included in the oral cavity through removal of the facial cyst wall, a procedure which Garretson had already described in a similar manner, but which seemed to him too involved and painful. Not until 1910 Partsch recommended the method, which he had previously rejected, of stripping smaller cysts of their follicles and suturing the wound immediately with silk thread. Both ways have stood the test to the present day; in German-speaking areas they are named in honor of the author, "Partsch I" and "Partsch II." The surgeon Partsch justifiably took credit for having pressed the scalpel into the dentist's hand.

Treatment of Fractures of the Jaw

Taking care of fractures of the jaw, the first diagnoses and prognoses of which are found in an Egyptian papyrus, lay unequivocally in the hands of the surgeons until after the middle of the 19th century. Particularly with regard to the mandible, it had hardly progressed at the end of the 18th century beyond the theories of Hippocrates and Celsus, Abulcasim and William of Saliceto: after resetting the teeth neighbored to the fracture line were joined by ligatures, and the corpus mandibulae was held immobile by a chin sling.

In the 18th century the capistrum was recommended by the Parisian surgeons Charles Gabriel Le Clerc and Jean Louis Petit as an aid to healing. While Le Clerc in 1700 used a "carton" formed to fit the chin, which was also done by Brun — schwig in 1497 and also by Heister in 1718, the famous Petit limited himself to bandages only in 1723. This was a generally observed regression during the 18th century and heedless of Hippocrates' warning against the dislocating affect of bandages. The illustration shows it in a slightly different manner. In 1788 Andreas Bonn in Amsterdam also represented typical maxillary and mandibular fractures in his atlas of bone diseases, but in his text there are neither the attempt to systematize nor any therapeutic recommendations.

Around the turn of the century the Parisian surgeons Chopart and Desault (1779), the Prussian regimental physician Rutenick (1799), the Englishman Francis Bush (1822) and the dentist of Braunschweig, Fr. Hartig (1830) constructed complicated, but in principle similar, apparatuses for the extra-oral fixation of the mandible.

The one by Rutenick consisted of splints from sheets of silver, wrapped in linen, which were laid over the rows of teeth at the site of the fracture and fastened under the chin by a hooked screw joint, with the help of a wooden plate like Le Clerc's "carton." He went beyond his colleagues in the use of a head cap for relief. According to contemporary reports (e.g. from Malgaigne) all of these apparatuses, despite numerous variations, could be worn only for a short period of time because of the sores they caused.

In his "Lecons sur les maladies des os" (Lectures on Diseases of the Bones), which

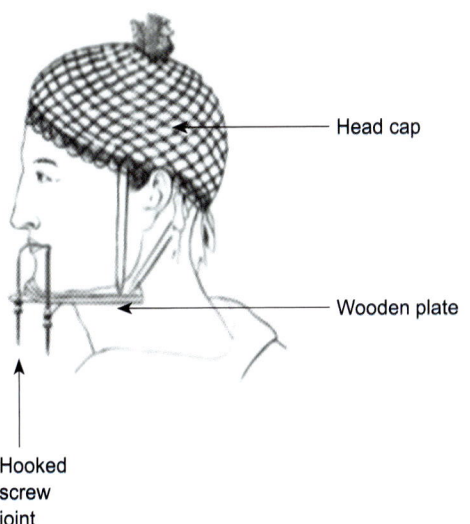

Fig. 3.4: The **apparatus for splinting a mandibular fracture** in place, 1799

was published in Paris in 1803, the surgeon Alexis Boyer recommended a kind of intraoral splinting. After application of the customary bandages he put particular emphasis on absolute immobility: An opening might also be preserved by introducing two pieces of corc, one on each side, between the teeth. Presumably the mandible was fixed in this situation by a capistrum. In 1836 the chief surgeon in Nurtingen, Wurttemberg, Johann Paul Spaeth, claimed that this material was too soft and smelled badly. Therefore he had a turner produce two doubly grooved horns for him, one for the sick and one for the healthy side.

In 1840 the military surgeon Jean-Baptiste Baudens presented in Paris the case of an oblique fracture of the corpus mandibulae, immobilized by threads brought through the skin on both sides of the bone with a needle and knotted over the crowns of the teeth, an anticipation of circumferential wiring. This Al-phonse Robert performed in Paris in 1852: he looped a silver wire over the row of teeth and over a lead plate (later zinc), which was lingually adapted to the teeth, and knotted it under the chin over a tampon. This way the wire served to hold the metal plate in place, and therefore only indirectly adjusted the fracture. An early wire suture, perhaps the first, between two holes drilled next to the fracture line was already publicized in 1847 by Gurdon Buck, a surgeon at the New York Hospital.

Victor Morel—Lavallee's methods were important for further development. In 1855 he advised after repositioning and immobilization by wire ligatures to press softened guttapercha over the row of teeth until the occlusal surfaces were covered by only a thin layer of it. In special cases he employed a kind of impression tray (moule) as an aid, which was fastened under the chin by a spring and a plate soldered to this. This method may have formed the basis for the later development of the hard rubber splints.

In 1855, the same year as Morel in Paris, Frank Hastings Hamilton of Buffalo, who was later a medical inspector during the Civil War, Informed the American Medical Association of a similar procedure. He softened two pieces gutta-percha and with them wrapped the back teeth on each side of the mouth; taking care, of course, that on the fractured side the splint extends sufficiently far forwards to traverse thoroughly the line of fracture. Thereupon he applied the four-tailed capistrum described by himself. Later, in 1857, he had a kind of impression tray (silver cap) made for him by a dentist, which he filled with gutta-percha.

The first mention of arrangements for maxillary fractures comes from the personal surgeon to three English kings. Richard Wiseman, in his case reports of 1676, "Severall chirurgicall treatises." This "British Pare" was called to a youth, his face being beaten in and the lower jaw sticking out from the blow of a hoof. He inserted his finger behind the uvula and pulled the body of the maxilla forward; when it was released, however, it immediately returned to its former position. Then, he formed an instrument bended up at one end, which he called my Extender, but the fractured body returned back again. Then Wiseman made an improved instrument, with which the fragment was held in place alternately by the hand of the Child, his Mother, and my Servants until callus had formed.

Treatment of a partial fracture of the maxilla was described probably for the first time in 1731 by the important Parisian surgeon, Henry-Fran-cois Le Dran: Four distal upper molars (he did not yet differentiate between molars and premolars) of an old man were tipped palatally with their alveoli when he was run over. The mandible was fractured in several places in the region of the chin. To secure the shaky maxillary fragment, Le Dran had the Dentiste du Roi (court dentist), Jean Francois Caperon, bind the four teeth still firm in their alveoli to a fifth tooth with slings of thread. After application of a chin cap the six mandibular anteriors were ligated similarly. As soon as ten to twelve days later, the thread ligatures fell away, but the fragments had become firm-an early example of dental and surgical cooperation.

In comparison with these rather primitive attempts, it was a significant advance when, in 1822, the Berlin surgeon Carl Ferdinand (von) Graefe-who also performed the first successful surgical closure of a palatal cleft in 1817-had his doctoral candidate, Reiche, describe an apparatus, which was similar to the Rutenick attachment on the head in another form to immobilize the fractured maxilla. An upholstered steel forehead band bore two adjustable arms to support the fragment in the correct position.

Morel-Lavallee modified his guttapercha methods also for the maxilla. Thereafter, in the second half of the century, one supported the fractured maxilla with a splint of hard rubber bearing two wire bars called "deer antlers". This was an application of the Kingsley apparatus from 1880, but for the maxilla. Later it was connected elastically with rubber bands to a head cap.

With regard to the taxonomy of maxillary fractures, two French surgeons are particularly deserving of credit. In 1866, Alphonse Guerin in Paris described the horizontal separation of the tooth-bearing portion of the maxilla without dislocation, which bears his name. Subsequently, in 1901, the surgeon Rene LeFort of Lille stated that the fracture without dislocation is the rule. This knowledge, which presumably had been responsible for the lack of interest until then in fractures of the middle third of the facial skeleton, he had gained from 35 cadaver heads which he had subjected to various traumas and, after maceration of the soft parts, dissected. He found chiefly in his investigations those typical weak lines which result in three principal groups of fractures on

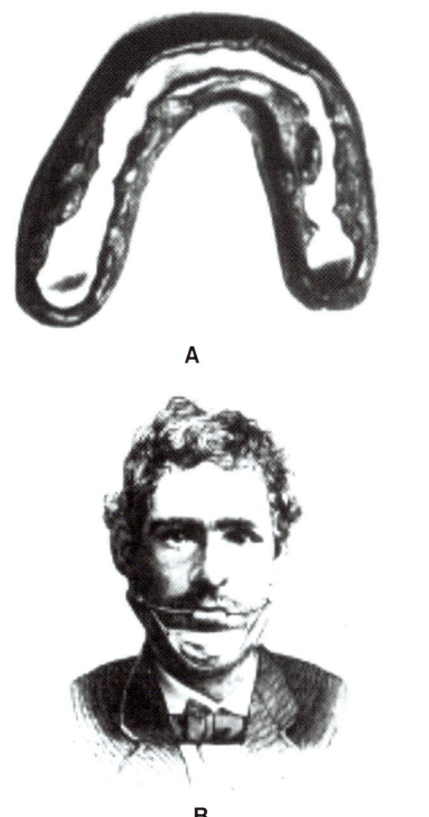

A

B

Fig. 3.5: Vulcanized rubber splint (A) and its **fixation by side bars** attached to a **chin bandage** (B)

the facial section of the skull and which still bear his name today.

In the dental textbooks of the first half of the 19th century jaw fractures are mentioned only peripherally as an incident in tooth extraction. If an author, such as Desirabode, devoted several pages to its therapy in 1843, the recommendations consisted only of quotations from surgeons, whereby Baudens' procedure was rejected as too painful.

The transfer of the treatment of jaw fracture into the hands of dentists took place in the second half of the century as a result of the use of hard rubber as a splinting material, which dentists in particular knew how to manipulate.

Its introduction in 1864 probably stems from two American dentists, the London-born Thomas Brian Gunning and James Baxter Bean. According to Gunning in New York, the mandible was first reduced and held in this position with wire loops so that an impression could be taken from both halves. A hard rubber splint enveloping both rows of teeth in the approximate position of occlusion was vulcanized from the models and fastened with screws to holes previously drilled in the molars of the mandible. The first patient treated after this principle was the author himself, who had been thrown from a horse. With regard to Bean the former Medical Inspektor Covey (in the defeated Confederate Army of the American Civil War, 1861–1865) reports that Bean had taken care of mandibular fractures in the last months of the war with an "interdental splint" of hard rubber. Bean took wax impressions of the single fragments, and placed the separated plaster casts in occlusion with the maxilla. The splint, which enveloped both maxilla and mandible, was held in place by a chin sling.

In 1881 a dentist in Quincy, Illinois, Thomas Lewis Gilmer who was later a co-founder of the Dental School at the Northwestern University in Chicago, reported on the fastening of "Gunning's splint" by twisting wire around the edentulous mandible, as had already been recommended in Paris by Robert in 1852. We also have to thank Gilmer for probably the first description of a percutaneous osteosynthesis: two pins were inserted in holes drilled next to the fracture line, and the two ends, the lingual one and the one protruding through the outer skin, were tied together with wire.

Even more important is Gilmer's suggestion of fastening the broken mandible to the maxilla. He treated a bilateral fracture first on one side by wire osteosynthesis and laced all remaining teeth of the maxilla and mandible singly with iron wire. The ends of each wire were brought together and twisted, fastening it securely to the teeth. This being done, the teeth of the lower jaw were exactly articulated with those of the upper and the wires of the lower teeth secured to those of the upper by bringing them together and twisting, thus firmly lashing the lower to the upper jaw. Herewith we have for the first time the reappearance of a method, which had already, been indicated but not actually described in an early print of William of Saliceto in the 15th century.

In 1865, at a dentist's meeting in Leipzig, J. H. C. Weber, a dentist working in Paris, was the first European to demonstrate a modified hard rubber dressing. He took an impression while trying to hold the fractured pieces in the best position. His splint comprised only the lower arch of teeth, the cutting edges and occlusal surfaces of which were left exposed, so that according to his statement, the patient was soon able to begin to chew (in contrast to the interdental splint), and complete healing seemed to have taken place after three weeks. Carl Haun, a dentist in Erfurt, proceeded according to the same principle in combination with guttapercha in 1867. In treating the wounded of the Franco-Prussian war (1870-1871), Suersen discovered Bean's impression method quite independently and presented it to his German colleagues in Berlin in 1871. He also had the idea of forcing apart mandibular fractures, which had healed with contraction by squeezing increasingly longer hickory pins between two hard rubber splints, which individually enclosed each fragment. Extra oral splinting of mandibular fractures was further developed in 1858 by Henry Hayward in London, who, after taking an impression, stamped an encircling metal plate and provided it with extraoral wire bars. This method was perfected by Kingsley in New York by the use of hard rubber plates, the upper sides of which he formed as occlusal surfaces. The bars were then held in place by a chin bandage.

Claude Martin, the Medecin-Dentiste and teacher at the Ecole du service de Sante militaire in Lyon, made special efforts towards further developing the encircling plate splint. Born on May 17, 1843 in St. Etienne as the son of a ribbon weaver Martin began as an apprentice to a lacemaker in Lyon. A dentist, struck by his adroitness, took him in as his apprentice and then sent him to Paris to his brother's practice. He was taken into lectures and clinical demonstrations by medical students whom he had befriended. Afterwards he studied for many more years under severe hardships in Paris and Lyon, where he settled as a dentist in 1873.

Leopold Ollier, the well-known surgeon, introduced him to the clinics where he took an interest in jaw fractures and especially in the field of surgical prosthetics. Here he advocated the necessity of an immediate insertion of the prosthesis, he had prepared for jaw resections (prosthese immediate), in order to counteract the traction by the scar tissue. He published his experiences, based on a considerable amount of clinical material, in 1889 in a comprehensive work in which he described the prosthetic reconstruction of the nose and other parts of the face, as well as the preparation of obturators.

Martin's method for splinting mandibular fractures, which he discussed in 1887 in a special book, was based on the principle of Morel-Laval-lee. He used hard rubber instead of guttapercha, and instead of the simple pelotte on the apparatus from 1855 he used a plate adjusted to the outer edge of the mandible, into which was fitted a steel spring. The outer plate bore hooks for rubber bands, which were fastened to a head cap, so that the splint and the upper arch of teeth were pressed against each other. He saw the advantage of this quite complicated apparatus in the fact that the patient could open his mouth to eat, an advantage, which was soon eliminated by the intramaxillary rubber lacing of the wire splints.

The first description of an arch bar as we know it today probably stemmed from the London dentist Gurnell E. Hammond, while working with the wounded in besieged Paris in 1871. He bent an iron wire on a model, which he passed over the teeth and fastened it with tying wire. This procedure was perfected independently by a method of the dentist Carl Sauer from Berlin who divided the bar, which was made preferably of spring-action gold wire, and joined it by lingually attached shells. The final reposition he left to the effects of spring forces, which proved particularly effective with older fractures where callus formation had already begun. In 1887 Sauer recommended soldering an inclined plane to the arch bar in the case of defective fractures and in 1889 he advised the use of an iron bar, adapted to the arch of teeth only on the labial side, as an emergency splint. It was bent previously by hand in the mouth to the ideal position, and the reduction was achieved through systematic tightening of the ligatures.

In the USA Angle attempted in 1890 to make his orthodontic system useful in the treatment of fractures; his procedure, however, was a step backwards because with the help of ligaments he rigidly tied the repositioned mandible to the maxilla, as Gilmer had done before. Heinrich Lohers, a dentist in Heidelberg, possibly stimulated by this method, used the ligaments for securing Sauer's arch bar with his own annular nut device in 1893.

It is difficult to ascertain by whom the intermaxillary traction with rubber rings, introduced into orthodontics by Tucker in 1852, was first applied to the treatment of fractures of the jaw. In German literature Karl Heitmuller in Gottingen recommended the application of an auxiliary bar to the maxilla in 1897, from which he pulled the depressed mandibular fragment into the occlusal position with rubber bands. Independently, in 1923, the dentist of the US Navy, W.L. Darnall, proposed the use of intermaxillary rubber bands for the first time in the United States.

Both of the systems whose evolutions are described here, the encircling plate and the tied-in arch bar, have undergone a parallel development in numerous variations up to the present time. The arch bar which could be produced without the help of a laboratory, proved particularly valuable in emergency cases and for military surgery. When nowadays the latter is enveloped by a cold-curing acrylic after being applied it means, in general, a union of both methods of treating jaw fractures in which the advantages of both are to a great extent preserved.

Increasingly, surgical (osteosynthetic) methods are being used today for difficult fractures.

REFERENCES AND BIBLIOGRAPHY

77. History of Dentistry by Walter Hoffman-Axthelm, 1981, Chapter 13, 326–358.

Chapter 4

Oral Surgery in the 20th Century

entistry today is somewhat specialized. The eight specialties include: Orthodontics, Oral Surgery, Periodontics, Prosthodontics, Pedodontics, Public Health Oral Pathology and Endodontics.[78] Maxillofacial surgery is a relatively young specialty of medicine and it was not established as an organized specialty until the second half of the 20th century. At first it was supported by general surgeons with particular interest in this field and also by inspired, extremely talented dentists. During the past few years modern techniques have brought decisive progress also in maxillofacial surgery, leading to rapid further development of diagnostic and therapeutic possibilities. The development of our specialty in the past century is discussed on the four main points of our scope, traumatology, orthognathic, cleft and tumor surgery.[79]

DENTOALVEOLAR SURGERY

The alveolus is that part of the bone of the jaw which supports the teeth and may be involved in any disease process affecting the teeth, jaws and surrounding structures. Dentoalveolar surgery, therefore, is the surgical management of diseases of the teeth and their supporting hard and soft tissues. It does not include

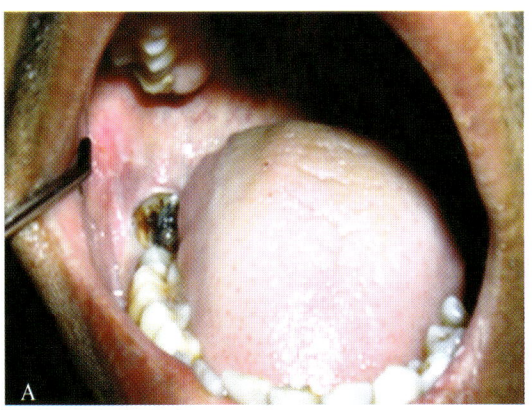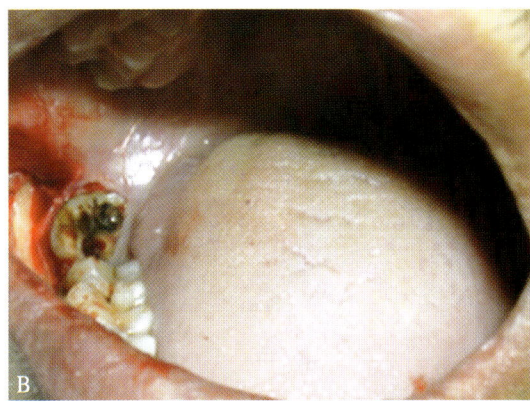

Fig. 4.1A and B: Depicting the surgical removal of mandibular third molar. (A) Preoperatively; (B) Incision and flap elevation

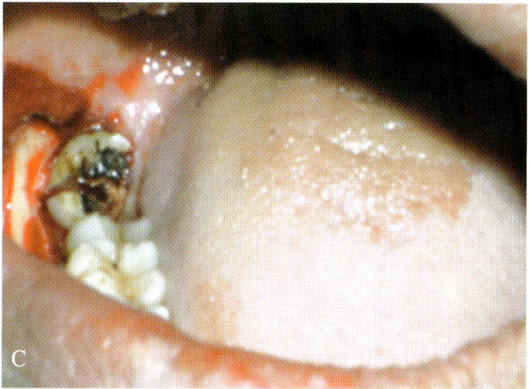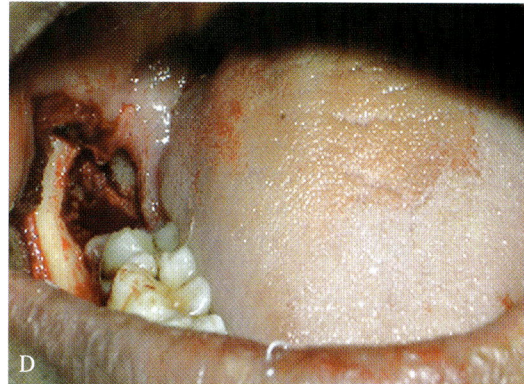

Fig. 4.1C and D: Depicting the surgical removal of mandibular third molar. (C) Tooth sectioning; (D) Extraction socket after complete tooth removal

dental surgery, i.e. the restoration of teeth and provision of crowns, bridges and other prostheses.

Impacted and ectopic (misplaced) teeth may result in a number of irreversible hard and soft tissue pathological conditions that can reach an advanced stage with minor or no symptoms, demanding a carefully balanced decision as to the timing of surgery.

The removal of impacted wisdom teeth is one of the commonest of all surgical procedures. The removal of impacted teeth, in most circumstances, can be carried out on a day stay basis, either under local anesthesia with or without intravenous sedation, or in designated Day Surgical Units under general anesthesia. Difficult impactions can be one of the most demanding procedures in maxillofacial surgery, carrying a significant risk of nerve injury and, without question; removal is most safely carried out by an experienced surgeon. In addition to the third molar, many other teeth have the potential for impaction, including pre-molar and canines and the expertise required to manage a full range of dentoalveolar presentations is considerable and remains a core activity of the specialty of oral and maxillofacial surgery.[80]

PRE-PROSTHETIC SURGERY AND DENTAL IMPLANTS

This is an important sub-specialty within dentoalveolar surgery and involves the restoration of oral and facial form and function that has been rendered deficient through loss or absence of teeth and progressive loss of related bony structures. A similar need may arise as a result of natural disease processes, trauma and surgery for tumors and related conditions.

The aim of pre-prosthetic surgery is to provide an environment for a prosthesis that will restore oral function, allowing normal mastication, speech and swallowing. By providing a stable and retentive prosthesis, gagging can be prevented along with reduction of pain and discomfort. This will also satisfy aesthetics and improve a sense of personal well being. Nowadays the scope and effectiveness of preprosthetic surgery has been extended by the application of endosteal dental implants alone or in combination with other surgical treatment, such as soft and hard tissue augmentation with grafts.

The endosteal implant is a device made of a biocompatible material, usually titanium, which is placed within bone and in time becomes directly attached to vital bone tissue, a process termed osseointegration. When placed within the jaw bone, implants can carry a fixture to provide anchorage for a dental prosthesis and they may also be placed into the skeleton of the face or skull to retain prosthesis such as artificial eyes, ears, noses or other missing parts of the face.[81]

HISTORICAL PERSPECTIVE

The first attempts by man to replace lost teeth with implants dates to the 18th century when it was common practice to replace lost teeth with the teeth of other individuals. These individuals were usually young boys or girls who were paid for their donation. The implantation of other individuals teeth met with resounding failure as the body's immune system quickly attacked the foreign tissue leading to infection and rejection of the tooth.

Early pioneers in implantology quickly realized that other inert material such as ivory or gold were not rejected as quickly. Even though these materials were an abhorrent failure as well, it took longer for the body to reject them. Implantologists went back to work experimenting with different metals. In 1891 a physician named Hartman proposed that dentures be fixed to the jaws using metal screws. Although a great number of failures quickly led to the demise of this procedure as well, the foundation was laid for the first crude, potentially successful dental implant system. In 1939 a dental clinician by the name of Stock attempted to alter the shape of the dental implant to resemble a wood screw. This ushered in a new era of dental implantology with multiple variations of Stock's initial work.

In spite of new materials and shapes, implant success was fleeting. Although the implant site healed, loading of the dental implant with a crown or bridge quickly led to loosening of the fixture, with infection and failure.[82]

It was during the early 1950's and 1960's that Per Ingvar' Branemark, beginning at the University of Lund and continuing at the University of Gottenburg in Sweden began researching the healing capabilities of the human body. One of his experiments involved the incorporation of two different types of metal cylinders into the jawbone of rabbits. These metal cylinders were implanted in the bones of the rabbits to determine how the body healed after injury. Dr. Branemark theorized that the only way to observe the healing process was to place small optical chambers inside the metal cylinders directly in the bone. He observed that, at the end of the experiment, the optical chambers housed in titanium metal would not come out. They had "fused to the bone". He coined the term for this fusion "osseointegration". He used this term to describe the reaction of the titanium to the bone. This term is still used today and describes the successful placement of the dental implant into the jaw.

On the basis of these experiments other trials followed. This culminated with the development of an implant system that could be surgically placed in the jaws, allowed to osseointegrate and then be restored with metal connectors to artificial teeth and modified dentures.

With a few modifications, Branemark's system of dental implants has evolved into the most successful implant system in use today. New sizes and better and more user-friendly components for the attachment teeth have been forthcoming.

Dental implants are used in the rehabilitation of patients following cancer surgery and can be inserted into bone grafts used to reconstruct the jaw, to allow artificial teeth to be worn to restore function. They can also help to retain obturators used to seal defects in the palate and have a role in the management of congenital abnormalities such as cleft lip and palate.

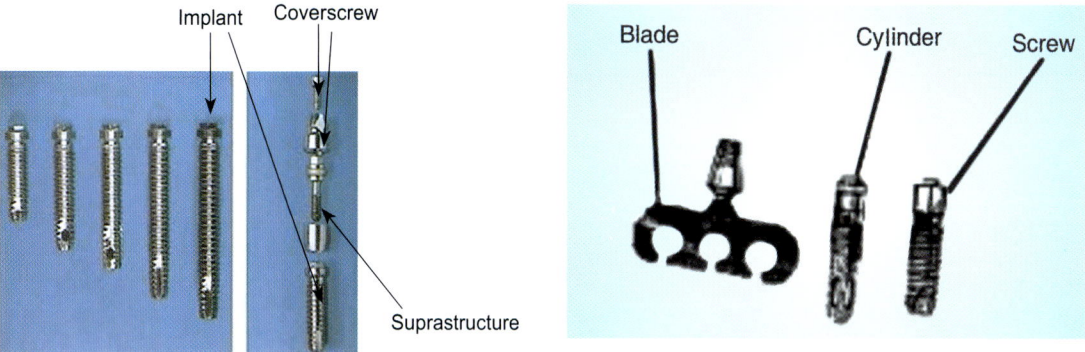

Fig. 4.2A and B: Branemark implant system (A) and 3 types of **endo-osseous implants (B)**

Patients who have lost teeth have sometimes been described as "oral cripples", unable to bite and chew effectively or speak clearly and in some cases totally unable to wear dentures. Such patients not only suffer physically, but they also suffer psychologically, becoming embarrassed in company and increasingly anxious, and in some instances become reclusive. The placement of dental implants has now been well proven to be highly predictable and developments in relation to immediate replacement of lost teeth and immediate or early loading of dental implants is transforming this field of practice. Once again, the oral and maxillofacial surgeon has an important role, particularly in the more complex cases requiring bone grafts and multiple fixture placement, and it is important that these treatments are provided within the context of a multi-disciplinary team including restorative dental surgeons and dental hygienists.

Because of the relative expense of treatment, there is a limited availability, but it is becoming increasingly apparent that the treatment of choice when teeth are lost is to replace the missing teeth with a prosthesis based on an osseo-integrated implant. In the long term it is possible that such treatment will be very cost effective.

MAXILLOFACIAL TRAUMATOLOGY

Advanced Trauma Life Support (ATLS) to accident victims is delivered by a multi-disciplinary team of which oral and maxillofacial surgeons are an inseparable part.

Injuries to the maxillofacial area are routinely treated by the technique of open reduction and internal fixation, using a variety of micro, mini and reconstruction plating systems. This has lead to early restoration of function and rapid rehabilitation, but there is no doubt that many serious facial injuries can cause permanent facial disfigurement and psychological distress with extensive soft tissue scarring presenting a particular challenge to the oral and maxillofacial surgeon.[83]

Traumatology has always been an important column and played a decisive role in the establishment of maxillofacial surgery as an independent specialty A retrospective of the past 100 years of traumatology starts with the conservative splinting of fractures of the upper and lower jaws and ends with the surgical treatment of panfacial fractures using

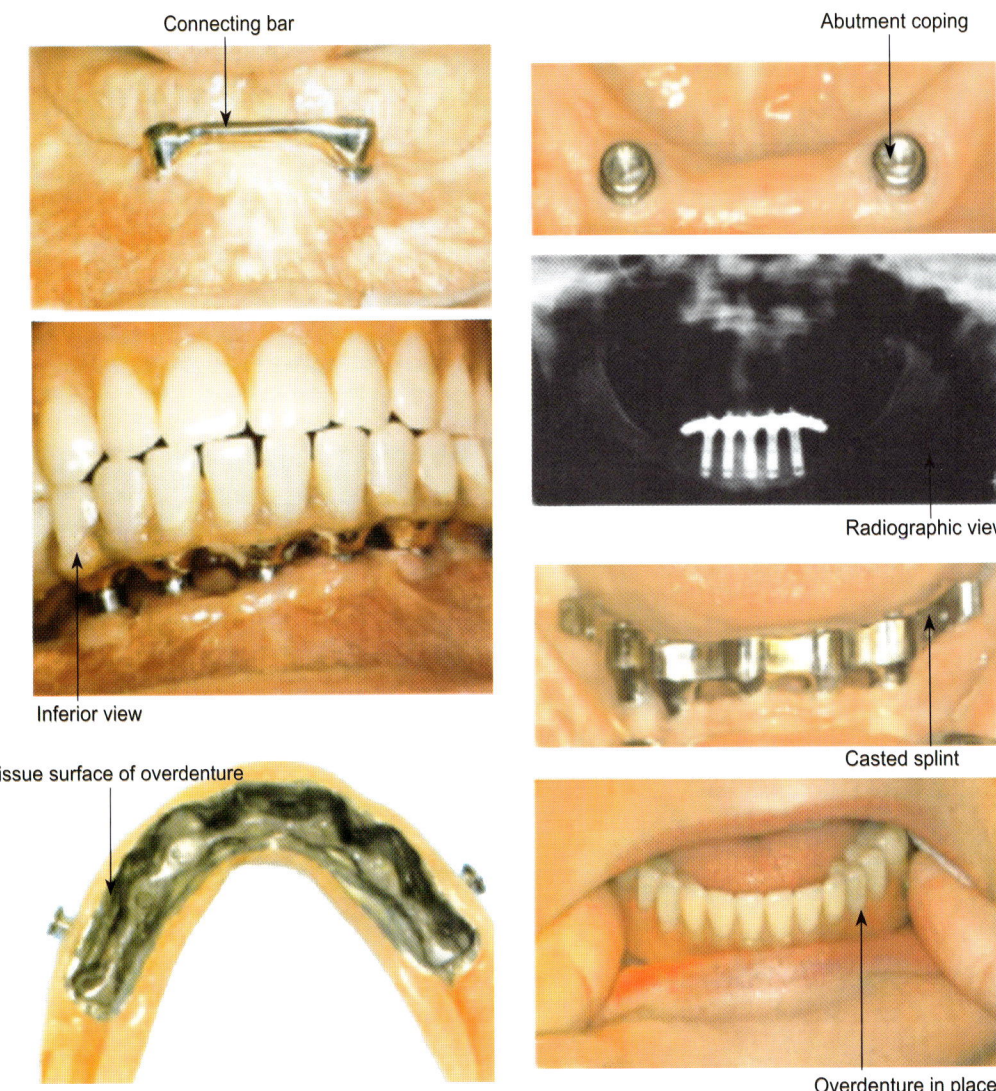

Connecting bar

Abutment coping

Radiographic view

Inferior view

Casted splint

Tissue surface of overdenture

Overdenture in place

Fig. 4.3: An **implant supported overdenture.**

plate osteosynthesis for internal fixation and the subtle repair of all structures of the facial skull.

In 1871 the London dentist Gurnell Hammond was the first to use an intraoral wiring in our present sense, and at least in Germany the continuous wiring technique is still called Hammond splint'. This classic conservative fracture treatment with rigid fixation of upper and lower jaw was modified many times, and again and again new types of splints were introduced over the years. In fractures of the upper jaw wiring was combined with extraoral devices, which in Germany is called 'Hirschgeweih' literally translated 'antlers'. The Berlin maxillofacial

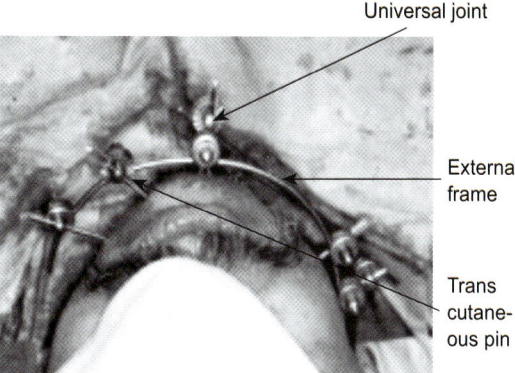

Fig. 4.4: Fixateur extreme (**external fixation**)

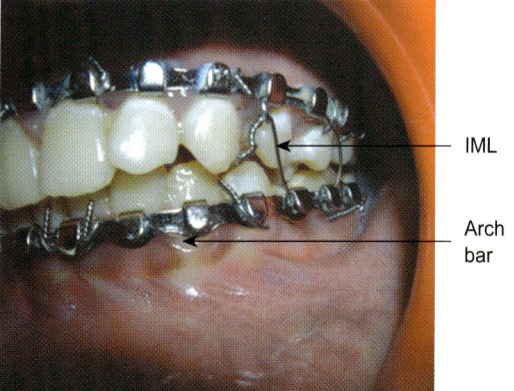

Fig. 4.5: **Closed reduction** for treatment of fracture

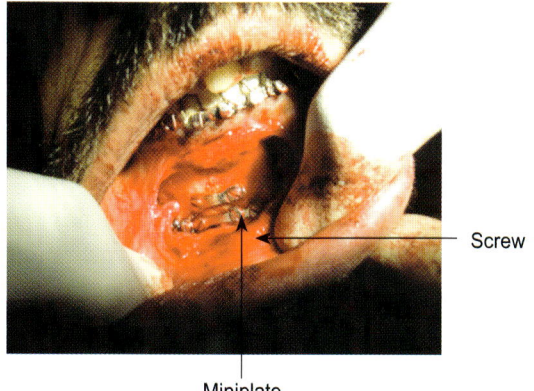

Fig. 4.6: **Mini plate osteosynthesis** for fracture mandible

surgeon Martin Wassmund who was the father of the most important German school of maxillofacial surgery, achieved perfection in this conservative treatment as outlined in his classical textbook of 1925 Frakturen and Luxationen des Gesichtsschadels (fracture and dislocations of the facial skull). This type of fracture treatment was the therapy of choice until not long ago.

In the thirties, attempts were made to stabilize lower jaw fractures by means of a 'fixateur externe' as we call it today.

In 1936, the Paris surgeon Grace George Ginestet developed the method, which had originally been invented by Roger Andersen (1963) for surgery of the extremities. Ginestet (1958) first presented it at a meeting of surgeons in Paris. He was very successful with this method, but the method was never fully accepted. However, it experienced a renaissance with the introduction of distraction osteogenesis.

The American maxillofacial surgeon William Milton Adams was the first to invent internal fixation for fractures of the upper jaw .In 1942 he used subcutaneous wires to fix the mobile fractured maxilla to the infraorbital margin. This technique soon was further developed in the form of fixation to either the zygomatic arch or the lateral orbital rim. When using this method, extraoral, mostly very unstable techniques of fixation could be abandoned. It was the first step towards the development of a systematic treatment regime resulting in surgically stable fracture fixation.

Modern traumatology started with the development of osteosynthesis, which was one of the major steps forward in cranio-maxillo facial surgery in the past 40 years. It meant not only a decisive improvement in the treatment of fractures but also in orthognathic surgery, treatment of craniofacial malformations and plastic and reconstructive bone surgery (Luhr 2000) In the conservative treatment of fractures, restoration of dental occlusion was the only point of reference. In many cases especially of extensive midfacial fractures this led to aesthetical disadvantages because the fractured bones healed in malposition (dishface). In contrast thereto modern fracture treatment using osteosynthesis plates and screws allowed, for the first time, three-dimensional skeletal repair of the entire facial skull.

In 1968 Hans Luhr was the first to introduce automatic compression plates into maxillofacial surgery. Eccentric holes in the plates and the use of screws with a conical head put into effect the principle of axial compression. Luhr himself and later on the Swiss AO group around Bernd Spiessl further developed the principles of compression plate osteosynthesis and standardized it to become a routine treatment of mandibular fractures (Luhr, 1968,1972; Spiessl et al. 1971).

On the basis of Michelet's and Moll's experience (1971) and following own biomechanical studies, Maxime Champy and Lodde developed their method of miniplate osteosynthesis and introduced it for the treatment of mandibular fractures in 1976. More recent biomechanical studies have led to the development of systems of microplates which arc used in non-load-bearing bones of midface and skull. Microplates enable us to relocate and stabilize even the smallest bony fragments.[84]

STEREOLITHOGRAPHY IN MAXILLOFACIAL SURGERY

Stereolithography is an industrial process which uses data generated from computer assisted design (CAD) to generate three-dimensional models. The data drives a laser over a bath of photosensitive resin that produces a series of stacked slices, which produce a accurate three-dimensional industrial prototype or model. This technique can be used by the maxillofacial surgeon to produce three-dimensional representations of facial bony structures using data from CT or MRI scans.

These so-called bio-models can be extremely useful in a number of particular clinical situations involving bony facial deformities, as this process allows the accurate visualization of the facial skeleton.

It is an invaluable aid to both the diagnosis and treatment planning of congenital, developmental and post-traumatic conditions affecting the facial region. In particular, it allows the maxillofacial surgeon to appreciate spatial displacements in all three dimensions and to make accurate measurement of the deformity.

The correction of post-traumatic or developmental facial asymmetry has always been difficult. Great accuracy is required to achieve a successful surgical result, due to the fact that facial deformity and asymmetry is often the result of relatively small magnitudes of bony displacement or deformity. The surgeon is then able to practice the surgery on the model, thereby allowing full appreciation of the osteotomy bone cuts required to achieve the desired results, together with any areas that may require augmentation with bone grafts.

Finally, the means of fixation of the realigned bony segments can be predicted. Valuable theatre time can be saved, by allowing the pre-operative of bone plates to be used for fixation on the "postoperative" bio-model that demonstrates the planned realignment of the facial bones. This technique also ensures there is surgical accuracy in achieving the planned outcome for the patient.

Stereolithographic bio-models can also allow the measurement of volume estimation of both bony structures for possible implantation and of bony cavities for reconstructive purposes. Stereolithography has been used in maxillofacial surgery in the following situations:

- Late reconstruction of complex bony facial trauma.
- The diagnosis of and planning of corrective surgery for congenital facial deformities.

Deficient area to be augmented

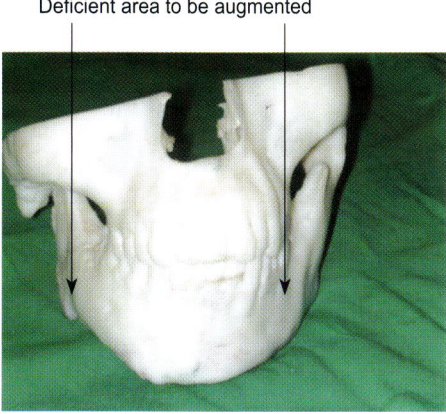

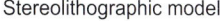

Stereolithographic model

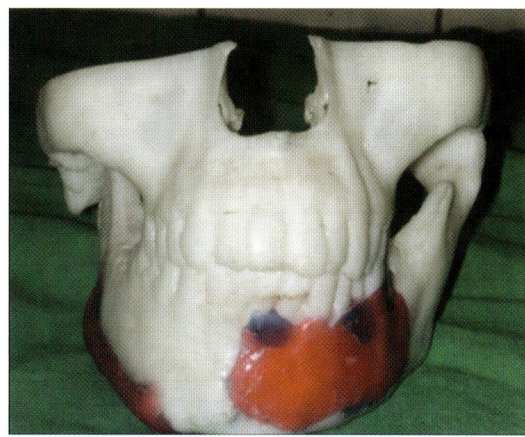

Planning done for augmentation on model

Fig. 4.7: Planning done for augmentation on a **stereolithographic model.**

- The diagnosis and planning of craniofacial deformity.
- Orbital volume estimation, for the correction of post-traumatic enophthalmos.
- Orbital reconstruction, following ablative surgery for malignancy.
- Evaluation of bone availability for the placement of osteo-integrated implants, both extra and intra oral.
- The pre-operative adaptation of temporomandibular joint prostheses for the treatment of advanced, degenerative joint disease, or post-traumatic bony ankylosis.[85]

THE TEMPOROMANDIBULAR JOINT

The oral and maxillofacial surgeon often plays a primary role in the diagnosis and management of patients with temporomandibular joint (TMJ) dysfunction. With several diseases affecting the joint and several imaging modalities available, the surgeon must decide which modalities are best for each individual patient. The goals of TMJ imaging are to evaluate the integrity and relationship of the hard and soft tissues, to determine the extent or progression of known disease, and to evaluate the effects of treatment. Diseases affecting the TMJ include various arthritis, internal derangement, developmental abnormalities, inflammatory conditions, and the effects of trauma such as fractures, dislocations, and ankylosis. All of these conditions can be evaluated with some type of imaging examination.

There are many ways to image the TMJ, from basic plain film radiographs and pantomography to sophisticated modalities such as computed tomography and magnetic resonance imaging. Other techniques, such as nuclear medicine and single-photon emission computed tomography (SPECT), have also been useful in the evaluation of the TMJ. Thermography has been used experimentally and may play a role in the diagnosis of joint inflammation, whereas ultrasound has been found to be of little value in TMJ imaging.

Basic tomography continues to play an important role in TMJ imaging. The role of CT scans is usually reserved for suspected tumors, foreign body reactions to implant materials, ankylosis, and trauma. Arthrography is a technique sensitive method for indirect visualization of disc position and morphology. With fluoroscopic imaging, joint movement can also be studied. MRI has provided an excellent, noninvasive method of assessing disc position

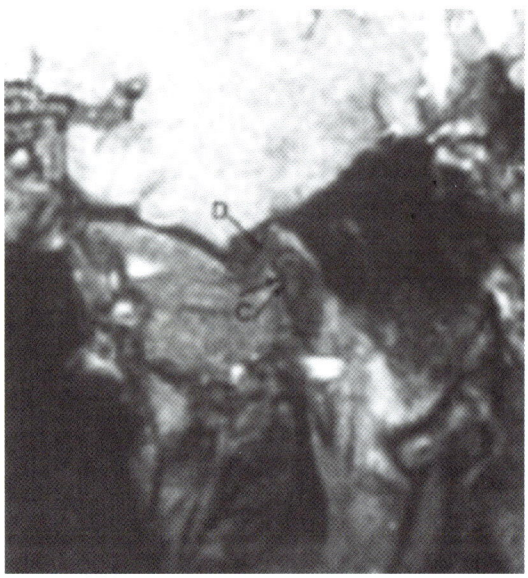

Fig. 4.8: Direct sagittal scan of TMJ MRI showing anterior displacement C-mandibular condyle D-disc.

and morphology. Although tomographic and CT images are still considered superior for the assessment of osseous structures, high field strength MR machines have shown good results in the evaluation of degenerative joint disease.

Ideally, the choice of imaging modality will depend on the patient's signs and symptoms. However, the decision will also be influenced by clinician experience, availability and access to equipment, and technical expertise. The best decision will be made by the clinician who is aware of the strengths and limitations of all the various modalities.

Once diagnosed the treatment may be either conservative or surgical. In the past, surgery for TMJ disease was less scientific and the results were appropriately variable, but now there is deeper understanding, better investigation and subspecialization of surgeons, which appears to improve outcome. Treatment is aimed at controlling inflammation and decreasing discomfort with anti-inflammatory drugs, including steroid injections, together with manipulation and physiotherapy etc. These patients are best managed by oral and maxillofacial surgeons with a special interest in these conditions.[86]

ORTHOGNATHIC SURGERY

"Surgery to create straight jaws" is the literal meaning of orthognathic surgery. Such corrections are largely achieved by osteotomies, surgical techniques by which parts of the jaw are cut to create separate fragments, which can then be moved into new positions with preservation of their blood supply.[87]

Orthognathic surgery is an original and a proper field of maxillofacial surgery. Since the time of our first teachers in the early 20th century the methods of orthognathic surgery have become more and more perfect. A large number of surgeons have concerned themselves with orthognathic surgery over the past 100 years so that there have been available many different operating techniques for the correction of skeletal dysgnathia of upper and lower jaw, the authorship of which were not always clear. It has been a long way until the presently performed combined therapy of orthodontic treatment and orthognathic surgery. In the beginning was the isolated correction of the lower jaw only. The first operation to correct a prognathic mandible by means of an ostectomy in the mandibular body was performed by Blair at the turn of the 19th century (1906).

Many modifications of this method followed. Today ostectomy in the mandibular body does not play any important role any more.

Lane from UK was the first to recommend sections of the mandibular ramus in order to correct mandibular prognathia. This was the beginning of osteotomies in the ascending ramus of the mandible. Unfortunately, Lane did not publish anything. In Germany, we connect osteotomies of the ascending ramus with the names of Lindemann (Lindemann and Hofrath, 1938) and Bruhn (1921), while in

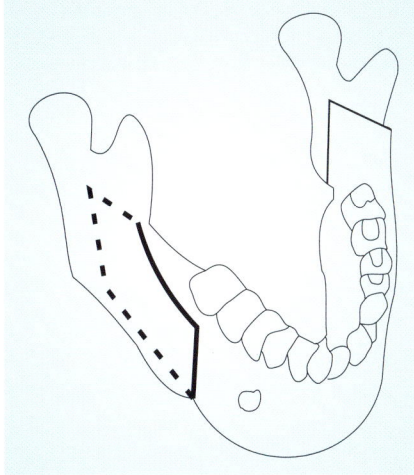

Fig. 4.9: Obwegesser's osteotomies of the ramus

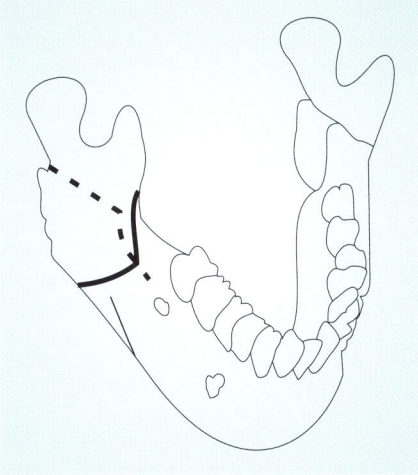

Fig. 4.10: Epker's modification of sagittal split ramus osteotomy.

the US literature this operation is dated back to Babcock (1909).

The breakthrough in prognathic surgery occurred when the method of sagittal splitting of the mandibular ramus was introduced by Trauner and Obwegessor in 1955. Hugo Obwegessor (1963) introduced the intraoral approach and thanks to him the method was brought to perfection and is now acknowledged worldwide as a standard technique. This was also the beginning of the final breakthrough for orthognathic surgery.

The first Le-Fort I osteotomy of the upper jaw goes back to Bernhard van Langenbeck in the second part of the 19th century (1859). This was the same Von Langenbeck who played an important role in the development of palatoplasty. In 1927, Martin Wassmund was the first to describe a maxillary osteotomy to correct posttraumatic malposition of the upper jaw. In 1934, George Axhausen was the first to perform a total mobilization of the maxilla. It was again thanks to Obwegesser (1965, 1969) that by describing exactly the surgical technique and presenting excellent surgical results maxillary osteotomies in the different Le-Fort planes have

become a standard procedure. Important basic research was done by William Bell in 1969. In his anatomical studies in monkeys new information was gained on the vascularization of the upper jaw. Such information led to the development of the down fracture technique in Le-Fort I osteotomics, which was the first step towards today's bimaxillary surgery. Without that maxillofacial surgery cannot exist anymore. Bruce Epker has also worked intensively in this field and presented many interesting suggestions regarding the planning and performance of orthognathic surgery (Epker et al, 1978).

While in former times the establishment of normal occlusion was the main guideline in orthognathic surgery, today, after the introduction of bimaxillary surgery, the major guideline is the patient's profile. In the past few years, the field of orthognathic surgery has further been supplemented by the introduction of distraction osteogenesis. In the early 20th century, experiments on the osteogenetic capacity or periosteum and endosteum in the lower and upper leg had already been performed, but the technique of distraction osteogenesis was acknowledged worldwide only after the publications of the Russian Ilizarov (1988).

As early as 1927 Wolfgang Rosenthal (1949) was the first to elongate the mandible in mandibular retrognathia by means of an intraoral distractor, a method that was then forgotten for many years. The first experimental studies of mandibular distraction were published by Snyder and coworkers in 1973. In 1992 McCarthy and coworkers reported his first four cases or mandibular distraction for correction of juvenile hemi facial microsomia after he had been inspired to this operation by Ilizarow's visit to New York in 1988. From this time on, the method has spread world wide and led to many technical modifications and the production of an abundance of distractors used today in many different cases. The technique of distraction is applied not only in mandibular anomalies but also in all kinds of defects of the face.

The surgical treatment or craniosynostoses also belongs to the surgery of malformation. The surgical rehabilitation of these malformations, which is, fully acknowledged today, was not established until the second half of the 20th century. Its interrelation between neuro- and viscerocranium had already been pointed out by Crouzon in 1912, but at the beginning of the century the therapy of craniosynostoses consisted only of strip-like ostectomy to reduce the intracranial pressure.

The decisive improvement was achieved through the pioneer work of Paul Tessier in 1967, who was the first to use the combination of an extra- and intracranial approach. He was also the first to conduct the fronto-orbital and midfacial advancement in elderly patients suffering from Crouzon's or Apert's syndromes. He developed the tongue-in-groove technique, the principle of which was based on the immediate molding of the malformation.[88]

CLEFT LIP, ALVEOLUS AND PALATE

Patients with clefts of lip, alveolus and palate are the largest group of patients with maxillofacial malformations. Clefts are very complex malformations affecting many structures that are all interdependent with each other. Cleft repair therefore requires a certain visionary quality of the surgeon. Until today it has not been possible to fully understand and analyze all phenomena of clefts. Ralph Millard had dedicated his life to the repair of cleft lips and palates and summarized his experience in three volumes of his fascinating textbook "Cleft Craft" (1976, 1977, 1980). He came to the following conclusion: cleft lips and palates are a never-ending challenge. This motto is still true for all our efforts in cleft surgery (Bitter, 2000). Therefore, here we will discuss only some very important milestones of cleft surgery over the past 100 years.

The basic principles of surgical closure of cleft lips and cleft palates were established as early as in the late 19th century. But only in the thirties of the 20th century Victor Veau, a pediatric surgeon from Paris, systematized cleft surgery and recognized that aspects of physiological growth needed to be taken into account in cleft surgery (Veau 1922, 1931, 1937).

In the surgical repair of cleft lips two different lines of incision have been advocated until today. The linear line of incision was applied by many surgeons and was still used by Veau and Blair in the early 20th century. The angular line of incision was introduced by Werner Hagedorn in the late 19th century (1884) and most of the recently applied more complicated lines of incision are based thereon.

Even today there is competition among the different methods according to Veau (1937), Millard (1976), Tennison (1952), Rendall (1959) and Pfeifer (1970 a and b) which are just modification of either the linear or the angular incision.

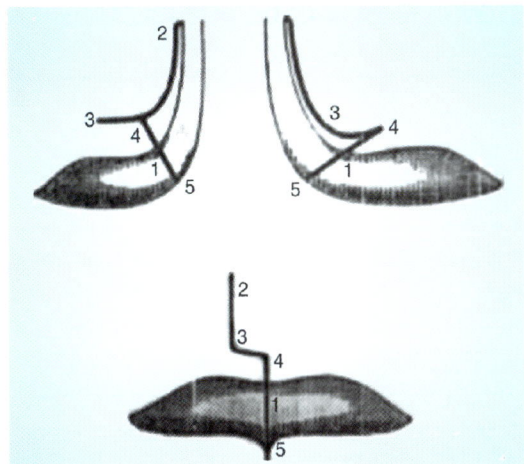

Fig. 4.11: Angular line of incision by **Hagedorn.**

Thanks to Jean DeLaire who reintroduced Veau's function oriented surgery, attention was called to the false muscular insertion in the region of midface and nose in patients with clefts of lip, alveolus and palate. Such deficiencies is impeding the normal development of nose and midface, especially of the bony structures. As a consequence Delaire (1975,1978) developed the principle of "functional closure" namely, the falsely inserting muscles were fixed to

the nasal septum thus aiming at establishing proper conditions for a physiological growth of the midface.

The surgical techniques of closing a cleft palate go back to the bridge flap introduced by Bernhart Von Langenbeck and the pedicle flap advocated by Veau (1922,1931). Closure of the hard palate was brought to perfection by Veau in that he was the first to repair also the nasal mucosa.

Anatomical studies made by Otto Kriens (1969) were of great importance for modern Veloplasty. Kriens found that the major pathophysiological criteria in velar clefts were dislocation and false insertion of musculature as well as absence of aponeurosis. He concluded that functional union of palatal muscles were successful only in terms of an intravelar myoplasty and construction of a closed muscular ring.

Another decisive step forward in cleft surgery was the principle of presurgical orthognathic repositioning introduced by McNeil in 1950 and later modified and further refined by Burston (1958) and Hotz (1964). A special type of preoperative treatment was developed by Latham in 1980 by means of a fixed intraoral device and its exactly defined

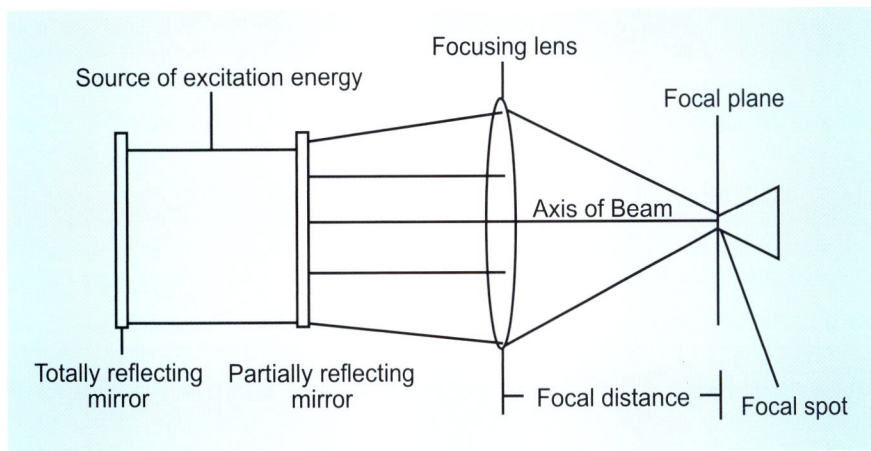

Fig. 4.12: The components of a laser.

forces that dislocated jaw segments of unilateral ad bilateral clefts were brought into a correct position within 3–4 weeks.[89]

MINIMALLY INVASIVE SURGERY— LASERS AND CRYOSURGERY

Both lasers and cryosurgery avoid the use of the scalpel and obviate the need for suturing. Certain laser wavelengths in the near and mid infrared can be taken down fibres into body cavities such as the temporomandibular joint, allowing a link with endoscopy. Excision of tissue by lasers is characterized by minimal scarring, for example of the oral mucosa, thought to be due to inhibition of myofibroblasts. Heat coagulation of tissue by penetrating laser wavelengths (e.g. Nd: YAG) and cold protein coagulation as by cryosurgery, leaves the body repair mechanisms to separate the devitalized tissue. In this process there tends to be a release of cytokines encouraging regeneration and an enhancement of local immune mechanisms.

Both lasers and cryosurgery have effects on nerve fibres, particularly the finer non-myelinated pain fibres, reducing pain by comparison with conventional surgery in general.

Lasers may be classified under the following headings:

High intensity laser therapy (HILT)—is used to cut or ablate tissue. For cutting a tissue a temperature of 100° C needs to be attained to boil the interstitial water, while for coagulation 60° C is necess1ary for full coagulation of proteins. Cutting abilities of lasers are most useful in mucosal subsurfaces for the removal of pre-malignant and early malignant lesions with minimal scarring, pain and tethering. The coagulating capabilities are best employed for vascular lesions such as cavernous haemangiomata. Care must be taken in the vicinity of nerves that will be damaged and cryosurgery can be combined with lasers to allow nerve regeneration.

Selective Laser Therapy (SELT): In this situation, one cellular population is selectively destroyed, leaving adjacent cells intact. There are two main methods:

(a) *Selective photothermolysis*: An example of which is the treatment of port wine stains of the face where a tunable dye laser may be used to produce yellow light in the 585 nanometer range. This will penetrate through the epidermis without significant absorption, to be taken up by the chromophore of oxyhaemoglobin in the capillary haemangioma, allowing selective damage to the intima.

(b) *Photodynamic therapy*: Which involves the administration of a light-sensitizing drug which is then activated by light, usually monochromatic (e.g. 630 nm helium neon laser). The interaction in the presence of oxygen precipitates cell killing. This photo-chemical reaction can be used to treat malignancy and pre-malignancy at a number of sites within the body. In terms of head and neck oncology a variety of photosensitizers have been used, each of which has different characteristics. For example, dysplasia can be managed using aminolaevulitic acid that produces a relatively superficial zone of tissue necrosis and leaves the patient photosensitive for a short period of only 24 hours. Healing is uneventful and takes place without any scarring.

Invasive tumors can be treated with a more powerful sensitiser, such as foscan which produces a depth of necrosis up to 1cm with surface illumination. This allows early invasive squamous carcinoma to be treated and the method is of particular use with field change disease and multifocal squamous cancer. In addition to surface illumination, photodynamic therapy can be carried out by intralesional implantation of laser fibres with up to four point sources being treated at one time, producing necrosis with a radius of about 1cm. The disadvantage of this treatment is that the patient may remain sensitive to light for about three weeks and, because of the more powerful nature of the effect, there does appear to be some postoperative scarring.

The only drug that is currently licensed for treatment on a world wide basis is photofrin which is a dihamatoporphyrin ether/ester mixture. This produces an intermediate range of necrosis down to about ½ cm with quite a prolonged period of photo-sensitivity, up to six-eight weeks. Healing takes place with virtually no scarring. It should be emphasized that at present, though this treatment offers great potential, the only routine services are being offered on study protocols.

Low Intensity Laser Therapy (LILT): Low power lasers in milliwatt ranges rather than the range of watts for HILT are used in the augmentation of healing, such as intractable orofacial ulcers, using a visible red light at 630 or 660 nm or near infrared irradiation around 830 nm singly or in combination, and in pain control. Using the near infrared irradiation of a gallium aluminium arsenide laser at 820–830 nm that penetrates at high energy densities, pain alleviation appears to be due to direct effects on fine nerve fibres, augmentation of cellular enzyme systems important in repair, and in some instances endorphin release.

Cryosurgery

For destruction of normal tissue, the attainment of a temperature of at least –15° C is necessary to produce intra-cellular ice formation, although for the destruction of malignant neoplasms –50° C is advocated. The normal ice ball shows the –2° C isotherm. The most potent method of freezing is by the use of phase change apparatus employing liquid nitrogen, where probes reach a temperature of approximately –180° C and a spray –198° C. Lesser potency may be obtained by the throttled gas method, classically employing nitrous oxide under pressure. In general, liquid nitrogen apparatus is indicated for the management of malignant disease and for lesions of bone, in view of its greater potency

of effect. The main uses for cryosurgery in the orofacial region are:

1. *Soft tissue ablation*: Cold necrosis may be produced in such lesions as hemangiomas or exophytic T1 carcinomas. Care should be taken in treating large areas of leukoplakia as a stimulant effect can be produced in peripheral zones.
2. *Pain control*: Temporary anesthesia may be produced for about 6 months by freezing peripheral branches of the trigeminal nerve, which may be useful in certain cases of trigeminal neuralgia.
3. *Bone may be frozen to remove residual aberrant tissue.* At least –15° C needs to be obtained and liquid nitrogen spray is most applicable to uneven bone cavities.

A pressure of between 8–10 lbs per square inch is indicated and cell ethal penetration occurs at a rate of approximately 3 mms per minute, i.e. about 3 minutes to freeze 1cm in depth. The method is particularly useful for keratocysts and benign neoplasms of bone, such as ameloblastoma. The lesion should be curetted and then freezing carried out for a suitable time, depending on the lesion.

If the mandible is already significantly weakened by tumor, there is a risk of pathological fracture in the third month after freezing, when re-modelling takes place. This can be offset by inserting a cancellous bone graft at the time of the original operation.

Both lasers and cryosurgery present a spectrum of exciting methods that result in a new concept of conservative surgery, augmentation and biomodulation. It is anticipated that they will find a special role in combination with gene therapy in the future, in relationship to orofacial malignant disease. Lasers lend themselves to gentle ablation of tissue with lack of bleeding and pain, while cryosurgery has special merits in relationship to nerve and bone that may regenerate after therapy. Both modalities of treatment are extremely important in the practice of oral and maxillofacial surgery.[90]

DISTRACTION OSTEOGENESIS

The ability to induce a callus in bone (by an osteotomy or sectioning) and then distract the proximal and distal ends is known as callatosis or distraction osteogenesis By performing an ostectomy on long bones Ilizarov, a Russian orthopedic surgeon was able to demonstrate that osteogenesis could be stimulated by distracting in a controlled manner the ostectomised bone. It relies on prolonged, progressive and gradual distraction that does not disrupt the vascular supply.

Principle

The osteotomy is usually carried out sub-periosteally and following this a latent period is allowed (usually 5 days) before beginning distraction. Distraction is achieved by fixators, which are attached directly to bone with plates and screws. At the end of the distraction period the bone should be allowed to consolidate under function into cortical and medullary phases.

Two main cellular processes are involved: the first is the formation of a callus and the second is generation of new bone by distraction. This technique has had a major impact in orthopedic surgery and is a developing technique in oral and maxillofacial surgery. The principal application of the technique is in the following situations:

1. Vertical bone distraction of the alveolar ridge in the preparation for the placement of intraoral dental implant fixtures
2. Distraction of the mandible by intraoral or extraoral distracters to produce lengthening, either in a jaw that has failed to develop (e.g., Treacher Collins) or in deformity produced by major trauma or as a result of tumor resection mid-face distraction in selected cases may produce significant advancement without the need for full surgical movement and the placement of bone grafts, by

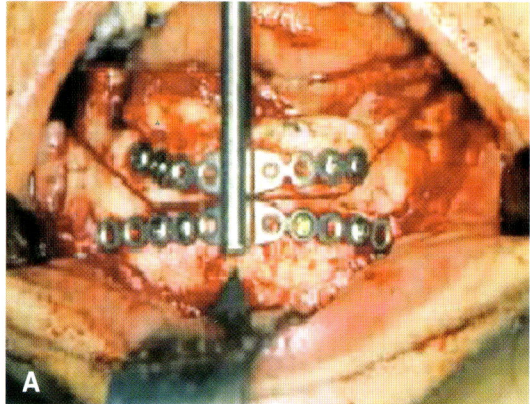

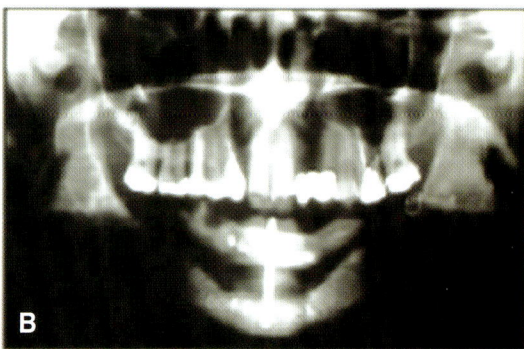

Fig. 4.13A and B: Distraction device (A) in place and post distraction CT revealing bone regeneration (B).

Percutaneous pins

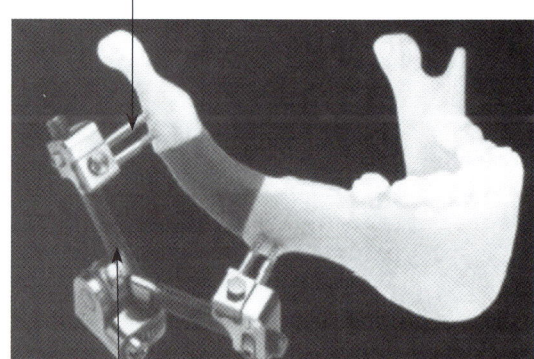

Bifocal external distractor

Fig. 4.14: A model demonstrating extra-oral distraction osteogenesis device for mandibular reconstruction.

distracting the mid-face from the cranium to correct craniofacial deformity.[91]

SALIVARY GLAND DISEASE

Saliva is essential for speech and swallowing and plays an important role in maintaining oral health by maintaining the integrity of the oral mucosa. It contains a variety of proteins with anti-bacterial activity and salts and minerals including fluoride and acts as a buffer and is, therefore, important in the control of dental caries and periodontal disease.

Salivary glands can be involved in many pathological processes, including congenital abnormalities, infections and other inflammatory disorders, obstruction, neoplasia and degenerative disorders. The most frequent problems seen in clinical practice are due to infections, obstruction from stones, benign and malignant tumors and destructive auto-immune disease. A specialist knowledge of dental and oral diseases is necessary for the proper management of these patients.

The management of salivary gland tumors requires specialized surgical skills due to the proximity of important cranial nerves and the often aggressive nature of the disease. Often patients will require a combination of surgery and radiotherapy to control their disease and should be managed on multidisciplinary clinics.

The salivary and lacrimal glands are subject to an autoimmune destructive condition, i.e. Sjögren's syndrome. It is often accompanied by other systemic diseases such as rheumatoid arthritis, systemic lupus erythematosis or primary biliary sclerosis. Patients develop severe oral symptoms relating to failure of salivary production and approximately 10% of patients with Sjögren's syndrome will develop a non-Hodgkin's lymphoma. These patients require meticulous follow-up in order to detect the onset of lymphoma at an early stage when treatment is still effective.[92]

FACIAL AESTHETIC SURGERY

Facial appearance is of the utmost social and psychological importance. There tend to be fairly standard ideals which constitutes a "normal" or beautiful/handsome face and many attempts have been made to quantify the proportions of the face and the produce the "ideal" face as a guide to artists and surgeons. Variations from the "norm" are often perceived as imperfections, or even outright ugliness by individuals who seek surgical correction. They are often self-conscious, lack confidence and may even be psychologically disturbed by their appearance. Other people may suffer an exaggerated ageing appearance which can be accelerated and accentuated by excess ultra-violet irradiation (photo-ageing), smoking, excess alcohol, diet or a combination of all four. Finally, and probably most importantly, faces can be disfigured as a result of facial injury or as a result of surgery for malignancy.

Facial aesthetic surgery is part of the training programme for higher surgical trainees in oral and maxillofacial surgery and as a specialty we have extensive knowledge of the growth, development, anatomy, function and inter-relationships of all components of the face and jaws. The most common procedures undertaken are as follows:

- Rhinoplasty, to alter the shape/size of the nose and to improve nasal function
- Pinnaplasty, to correct the fairly common deformity of "bat ears"
- Genioplasty, to correct deformity of the chin
- The ageing face, where the muscles start to sag, causing the overlying skin to sag also. This causes lines, grooves and wrinkles to appear. The problem can be improved by many procedures, including forehead lift, blepharoplasty ("eye bag" removal), rhytidectomy (face lift), cheiloplasty, where lips can be re-shaped with or without fillers such as collagen, Gortex strips or fat transfers. Skin texture and appearance can be improved by topical application of vitamin A

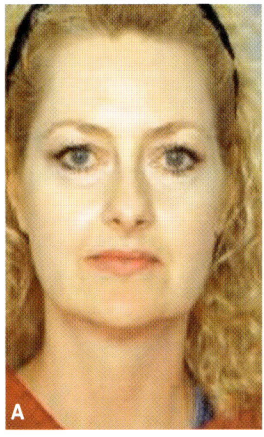
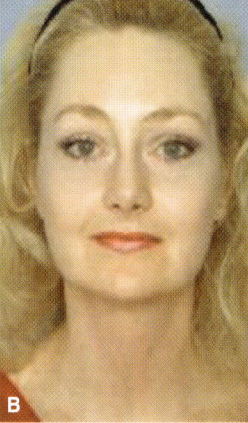
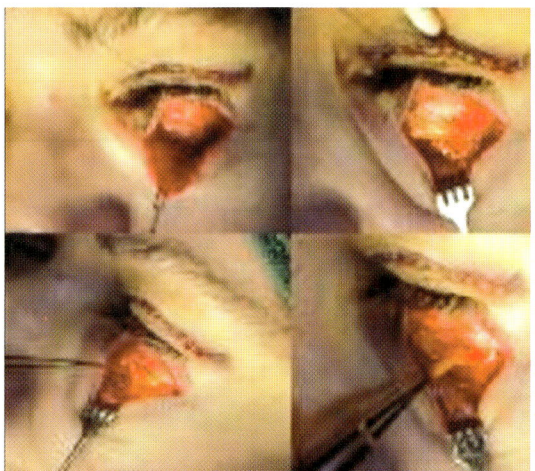

Fig.4.15A and B: Depicting the results of **Rhytidectomy**—Preoperative (A) and postoperative (B) appearances.

related components, chemical peels or laser skin resurfacing.

The latest chemicals include fruit acids. Acne scars can also be improved by these techniques and collagen can be injected as a filler for wrinkles, depressed scars and thin lips. The results can be quite good, although may be temporary and require frequent repeat treatment sessions.

In addition, the techniques of orthognathic surgery can vastly improve facial appearance and function and overall well-being and can be done in combination with facial aesthetic procedures.[93, 94]

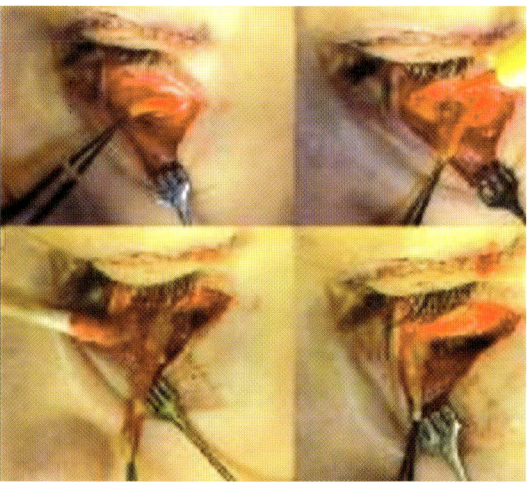

Fig.4.16: Depicting the surgical procedure of lower eyelid blepharoplasty.

OROFACIAL CANCER AND RECONSTRUCTIVE SURGERY

Maxillofacial surgery has considerably contributed to the development of surgical techniques for the treatment of head and neck tumors. This field of our specialty has been characterized by a rapid progress in the past 30 years, although we must admit that it has not been possible to significantly improve the survival rates for oral cancer patients. In this retrospective I will discuss only the surgical aspects of tumor surgery.

In the 19th century outstanding surgeons already dared to resect tumors from maxilla, mandible, tongue and lower lip and described operations which from our present viewpoint appear extremely heroic (Dupuytren, 1812;. Graefe, 1822; Gensoul, 1827; Dieffenbach, 1845, Weber, 1866; Von Langenbeck, 1875). Our present principle of tumor surgery in the oral cavity, namely 'wide resection of the primary tumor with a large safety margin and radical resection of the regional cervical lymph nodes'

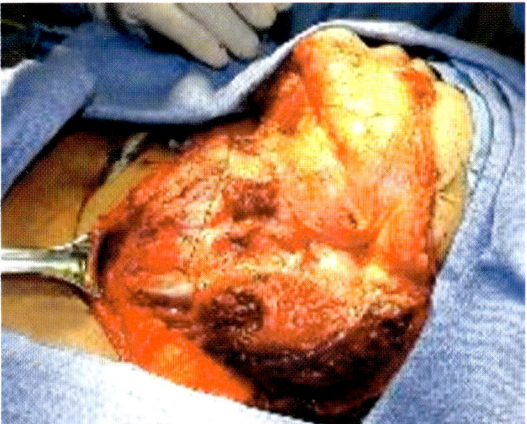

Fig. 4.17: Radical neck dissection

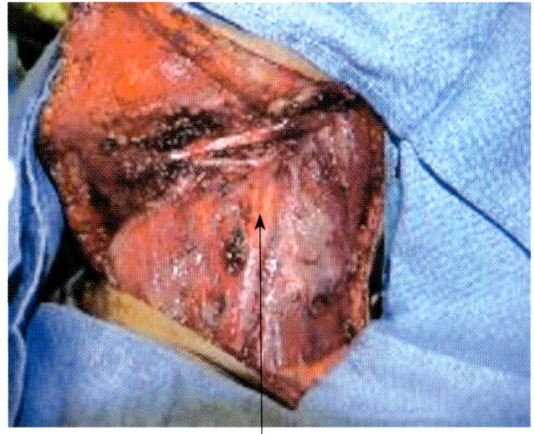

Internal jugular vein

Mucoperiosteal flap reflected

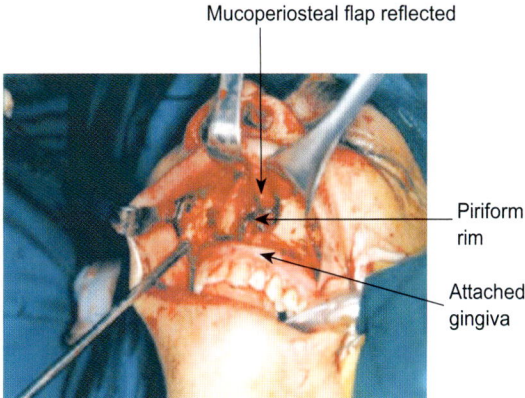

Piriform rim

Attached gingiva

Fig. 4.18: Midface degloving to access tumour of maxilla

was first established by Crile who presented this principle or block dissection at the 57th Annual Session of the American Medical Association in 1906. It was published in the *Journal of the American Medical Association*. The great importance of the publication of this classic surgical procedure is demonstrated by the fact that in 1987 the article was reprinted in its original version as a landmark article in the *Journal of American Medical Association*.

Following Crile, many different operating techniques and new ways or access to the tumors often hidden in the facial skull and difficult to reach have been described over the past years. Small intraoral T1 tumors can easily be exposed and resected via a transoral access. Tumors having deeply infiltrated the musculature of the tongue or the floor of the mouth require either a bilateral submandibular approach in form of a pull-through operation or a transmandibular approach with temporary section of the lip and osteotomy of the mandibular body (Boyle and Shah 1999).

In maxillary resections, the method of midfacial degloving introduced by Cason and co-workers in 1974 has largely replaced the Dieffenbach-Weber incision developed in the 19th century. Midfacial degloving means that the midfacial soft tissue is loosened from the maxilla and nasal skeleton using an intraoral and transnasal incision, allowing a good survey of the entire maxilla and the nasal and ethmoidal region without producing visible scars in the face.

The systematic development of skull base surgery also offers new perspectives and means a widening of the range of facial tumor surgery. In the sixties all specialties interested in the skull base founded a new association and maxillofacial surgery played an important role since it provided access to the skull base.

In 1985, Obwegesser described the temporal approach for the resection of tumors in the

Supraorbital margin   Marking for access osteotomy

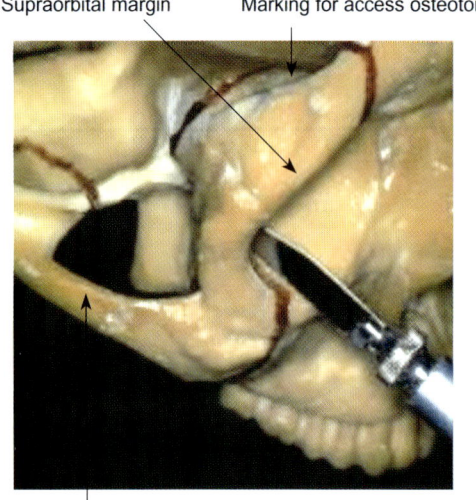

Zygomatic arch

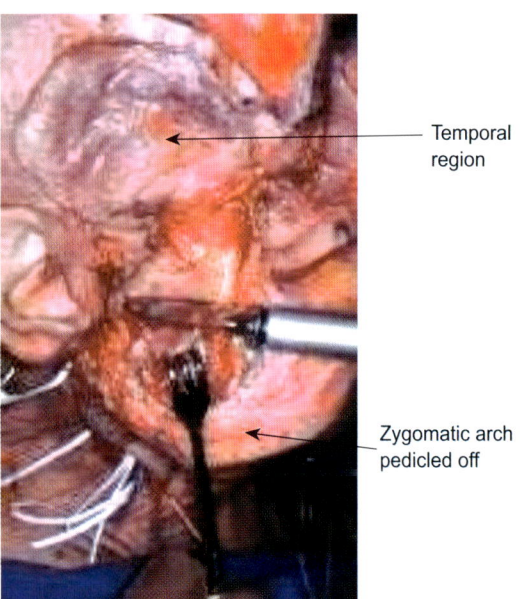

Temporal region

Zygomatic arch pedicled off

Fig. 4.19: Depicting infratemporal access for skull base tumours—an example of ***access osteotomy***

lateral part of the medial cranial base. Zygoma and zygomatic complex pedicled at the masseter muscle are displaced caudally and the ascending mandibular ramus pedicled at the temporal muscle is displaced cranially, thus widely opening the retro maxillary region. The

frontal approach to the retromaxillary region and the cranial base is across the facial skull, either through the midface or through the mandible (Curioni, 1989).

In cranio-maxillofacial surgery it is not possible to discuss tumor surgery without considering reconstructive surgery. Many radical resections of extensive malignant tumors of unfavorable location were made possible only following important progress in plastic and reconstructive surgery. Around 1920, Ganzer (1917), Gillies (1920) and Filatow (1922) introduced the tubed flap which was a breakthrough for the repair of extensive intra- and extraoral soft tissue defects. Tubed flaps meant long-term treatment. Consequently, this technique was applied only in secondary reconstruction and was the therapy of choice until the sixties and the seventies (Schuchardt, 1944).

The introduction of the acromiopectoral flap by Bakamian in 1965 and of more types of pedicled arterial skin and fat flaps a little later meant a quantum leap for maxillofacial surgery.

For the first time, those flaps made available high-quality soft tissue that could immediately be used for primary defect covering. With the development of the various pedicled myocutaneous flaps in the late seventies a change

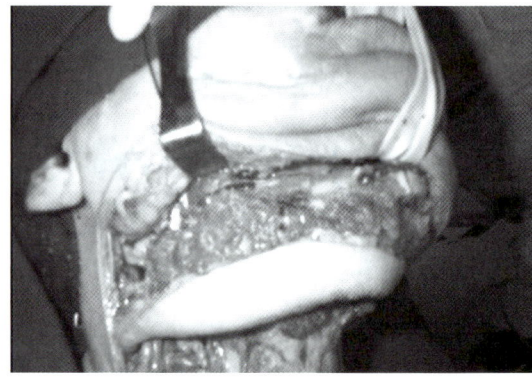

Fig. 4.20: Fibula osteocutaneous free flap reconstruction of hemimandibular defect.

from secondary to primary reconstruction took place, since primary repair of extensive intra and extraoral soft tissue defects became possible The introduction of the operating microscope into vascular surgery and the development or microsurgically revascularized free flaps meant another quantum leap and led to the methods of primary reconstruction that are generally applied today (Taylor and Daniel, 1975; Watson et al, 1979; Pennington et al, 1980; Nassif et al, 1982; Hausamen and Schneider, 1988).

In this connection it is important to mention that jejunal graft was introduced into maxillofacial surgery by Reuther and Steinau in 1980. Jejunal grafts were used to replace oral mucosa for many years. For the first time, this graft made it possible to repair extensive mucosal defects with a high-quality functional replacement.

Jejunal grafts are no longer the first-choice method in our department. We prefer the use of cutaneous flaps from the lower or upper arm, because they are taken more easily and produce less donor site morbidity. Nevertheless, it was thanks to Jurgen Reuther that microvascular surgery was introduced into maxillofacial surgery and only on the basis of microsurgery is it possible today to ensure postoperative rehabilitation with an acceptable quality of life for our patients.

In the 19th century defects of the bony structures of the face were restored by the use of prostheses covering the defect; this was particularly true for the mandible. In 1908 Georg Axhausen published his landmark paper on free bone grafting and thus laid the foundations for osteoplastic repair of the facial skull. Although the first bone graft to the mandible was performed by Sykoff (1900) a surgeon from Moscow, it was Lexer who systematically repaired mandibular defects with tibial grafts since 1907 and later used free grafts from the iliac crest for large defects. He described this method in his textbook Die

freien Transplantationen (The free grafts) that was published in 1924 and became the standard work of plastic surgery. Since then the technique of bone grafting has remained the method of choice for the replacement of the parts of the facial skull, only some variations have been introduced primarily with regard to fixing methods.[95]

CRANIOFACIAL SURGERY

Craniofacial surgery is concerned with the management of patients presenting with congenital or acquired conditions, affecting the hard and soft tissues of the head and face. Examples are:
- Craniosynostoses
- Craniofacial dysostoses
- Orbital dysostosis
- Encephalocoeles
- Craniofacial clefts.

These conditions are evident early in life and most patients are children under the age of 2. Patients referred to designated units are assessed and investigated by a multidisciplinary team and treatment combines the principles of maxillofacial reconstruction with neurosurgery. The surgical techniques employed in congenital conditions can also be applied to good effect in the treatment of skull base tumors and craniofacial trauma. Premature fusion of one or more skull sutures (craniosynostosis) occurs in 1 in 2,000 of the population. Syndromic craniosynostoses, such as Crouzon and Apert syndromes occur in 1 in 10,000 and 1 in 150,000 live births respectively. Facial clefts are even rare.

Historically, patients underwent numerous procedures performed by various clinicians from different surgical specialties. Results were generally poor and associated with high morbidity and even mortality. Many patients with severe deformity were denied surgery, because of the risks involved. In the 1960's, Paul Tessier showed that facial surgery could be safely combined with neurosurgery.

Craniofacial surgery was born and has continued to evolve. The surgery is major, often protracted and associated with significant blood loss in the small child. Intensive care is needed for the more complex cases, or where the airway is compromised. Some children require more than one procedure as growth and dental development influence facial form and function. However, with an active, established team and utilizing contemporary techniques, such as distraction osteogenesis, it is possible to perform fewer, more extensive procedures. The results are better and there are fewer complications.

The craniofacial principles of wide surgical exposure, primary bone grafting and internal fixation should be applied to the management of complex craniofacial trauma. Severely injured patients of all ages can be stabilized and offered early definitive treatment using these techniques. Morbidity is reduced and hospital stay shortened and there is an overall improvement in outcome. These surgical approaches can also be used to access intracranial and skull base lesions.

The management of craniofacial patients requires a collaborative and multidisciplinary approach if optimal results are to be achieved and the core disciplines are usually maxillofacial, plastic and neurosurgery, supported by anesthetic, ENT, ophthalmic and specialist nursing colleagues. By drawing on expertise gained in the management of trauma, tumor and congenital disease of the soft and hard tissues of the face, the maxillofacial surgeon plays a key role in craniofacial surgery. [96]

REFERENCES AND BIBLIOGRAPHY

78. History of Dentistry 2001 by Terry Wilwerding 4.
79, 84, 88, 89, 94, 95. "The scientific development of maxillofacial surgery in the 20th century and an outlook into the future"-an article from Journal of Craniomaxillofacial Surgery: 2001;Feb 29 (1); Pg 2–21.

80, 81, 83, 85, 86, 87, 90, 91, 92, 93, 96. History of British Association of Oral and Maxillofacial Surgery from the web.

82. "Who is a candidate for dental implants" –an article from the web.

Chapter 5

The Current Scenario in Maxillofacial Surgery

This is surely one of the great eras in our history for the practice of oral and maxillofacial surgery. We have achieved an enviable scope of practice. We have controlled the cost of the patient care and maintained access to care at reasonable cost. We have evolved from the crudest remedial measures that were being utilized at the grass root level, to the most sophisticated of the techniques thus increasing our efficiency and also rendering quality care to the masses. We have already seen how and when the various surgical procedures came into existence and that later underwent various modifications as per the need. Here we have a brief mention of the latest advancements and techniques that are available at present that has upgraded the specialty of oral and maxillofacial surgery.[97]

TRAUMATOLOGY

Modern oral and maxillofacial surgical techniques have resulted in early restoration of function and return to work and have reduced the need for secondary reconstruction and scar revisions. In collaboration with neurosurgical colleagues, it has now become possible for simultaneous management of severe cranio-maxillofacial trauma to be dealt with in a single stage, often using a shared surgical access.

The use of advanced imaging techniques such as CT scan, MRI and stereolithography are used to demonstrate the pattern of cranial and facial bony injuries and to plan better primary treatment.

Today open fracture reduction and the use of miniplate osteosynthesis is the state of the art worldwide and has proudly changed our thinking and understanding regarding the treatment of maxillofacial trauma cases. Modern treatment of midfacial fractures already starts with the type of approach to the operating field. In previous years we used mostly local incisions to enable surgical reduction. Such incisions allowed only a keyhole view of the actual fracture. Today open reduction of all bony fragments is performed in all fractures, which requires particular ways of access. We preferably use the bicoronal approach in extensive fractures of the midface sometimes combined with a mid-palpebral incision or an intra oral incision.

Joe Gruss (1987) and Paul Manson and his group (1985) have worked particularly in the field of midfacial and panfacial fractures and concerned themselves with the treatment of such fractures. They have taught us that it is especially important to stabilize buttresses of the facial skull with miniplates. Surgical repair of extensively comminuted fractures should start with restoring the zygomatic arches and the malar prominences as the major vertical and horizontal buttresses of the face by means of miniplates using a bicoronal approach. The restored lateral orbital rims and zygomatic arches will serve as an outer frame for the face. Then correct reduction of orbital, nasoethmoidal and frontal bone fragments and fixation by microplates is possible. Such procedure allows perfect reconstruction of face and cranium.

The modern principle of facial repair calls for primary reconstruction in the case of bony defects also in order to prevent shrinkage of soft tissue lining resulting from the loss of bony support. As primary bone grafts we normally use split calvarial bone grafts which can easily be harvested when using the bicoronal incision or by an additional coronal incision.

The formulation of resorbable implants made of polymers (such as polydioxanone, poly-glycolic acid and polylactic acid) for the osteo-synthesis of facial fractures has revolutionized the field of oral and maxillofacial surgery. The major advantage is that they provide adequate fixation for direct bone healing, but as the bone gains strength, the plate is gradually resorbed by the body. Although it has avoided a second surgical procedure for removal of the implant, but there are other problems inherent in their use that includes lack of material strength. Further research is needed in this direction.[98]

ORTHOGNATHIC SURGERY

The surgical treatment of craniosynostoses belongs to the surgery of malformation. The surgical rehabilitation of these malformations, which is, fully acknowledged today, was not established until the second half of the 20th century. Its interrelation between neuro- and viscerocranium had already been pointed out by Crouzon in 1912, but at the beginning of the century the therapy of craniosynostoses

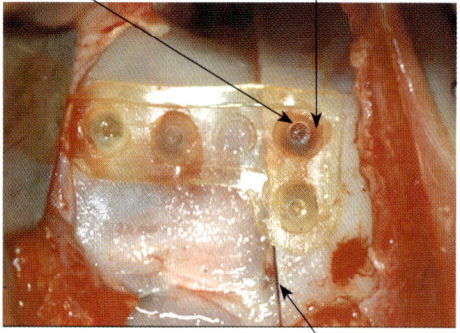

Bioresorbable screw   Bioresorbable implant

Osteotomy site

Fig. 5.1: Maxillary osteotomy fixed with a **Resorbable Implant.**

consisted only of strip-like ostectomy to reduce the intracranial pressure. Paul Tessier in 1967 was the first to use the combination of an extra- and intracranial approach. He was also the first to conduct the fronto-orbital and midfacial advancement in elderly patients suffering from Crouzon's or Apert's syndromes.

The present surgical procedures are based on this concept of advancement of the viscerocranium as a whole and so Tessier is considered as the father of craniofacial surgery.

A further progress occurred when in 1978; Daniel Macharc introduced the bilateral advancement technique in early childhood for the first time. This has resulted in decisive improvements of function and aesthetics, especially in extreme growth disturbances. Today, the fronto-orbital advancement is considered to be the safest basic method for the treatment of pre-mature cranial suture synostosis. Although craniofacial surgery is not exclusively a field of maxillofacial surgery, maxillofacial surgeons had a, substantial influence on the development of the therapeutic principles. Among the German-speaking colleagues Hugo Obwegesser and his work for the surgical interventions in adults and Jochen Muhling for the treatment of small children have to be quoted (Muhling et al, 1984; Muhling, 2000) in this respect.

While in former times the establishment of normal occlusion was the main guideline in orthognathic surgery, today, after the introduction of bimaxillary surgery, the major guideline is the patient's profile. In the past few years, the field of orthognathic surgery has further been supplemented by the introduction of distraction osteogenesis.[99]

CLEFT LIP, ALVEOLUS AND PALATE

Preoperative orthognathic treatment is generally accepted today and is applied in a modified form in all cases of complete clefts of lip, alveolus and palate.

Bone grafting to close the alveolar cleft is another important method of orthognathic treatment. The first bone grafts were tried in the beginning of the 20th century, but unfortunately their development first lead into a cul-de-sac. In 1926 Hans Pichler recommended the graftings of bone to close alveolar clefts. As a consequence so called primary bone grafting performed at the same time when closing the cleft lip that is in babies was applied in the 50s and 60s following research done by Stellmach (1955, 1963), Schmid (1955), Nordin and Johanson (1955) and Johanson and Omisson (1961). However, in the late 60s long-term follow ups showed that primary bone grafting was the wrong way, as it frequently impeded normal development of the upper jaw.

Our present state of the art of closing the alveolar cleft goes back to Boyne and Sands who in 1972 introduced a combination of orthognathic therapy and surgery: at the age of 9–11 years secondary bone grafting is performed, namely vital cancellous bone is transorally grafted to the alveolar cleft. Thus a bony area is created allowing spontaneous eruption of teeth adjacent to the cleft or their orthodontic treatment. Today metric accuracy is still a target of the future of cleft surgery and the different cleft centers vary considerably in their therapies. However cleft surgery in the 20th century has turned into an all round treatment allowing good rehabilitation of cleft patients due to the good cooperation among the different specialties ensuring a well balanced conservative as well as surgical treatment protocol. Cleft centers comprising all departments involving in cleft treatment are the real step forward in cleft treatment.[100]

CANCER AND RECONSTRUCTIVE SURGERY

Even the classic procedure for surgery of oral cancer has changed in the recent years. While block dissection as described by Crile in 1906 is still being applied today, Crile's concept of radical neck dissection has changed. Today a more conservative treatment saving the accessory nerve, internal jugular vein and sternocleidomastoid muscle is favored (Suarez, 1963; Bocca, 1966; Shah, 1990; Boyle and Shah. 1999).

In the German speaking countries the change in the therapeutical concept was brought about by DOSAK, the German, Austrian, Swiss Working Group for tumors in the maxillofacial region, which organized a therapeutical study on radical neck dissection versus conservative neck dissection in 1982. The results of that study revealed that so far life table analyses did not show any statistical significant differences between the two surgical measures (Bier et al, 1992; Schlums et al, 1992)

The microvascularly anastomosed bone graft is the only real novelty in the field of bone grafting (Taylor et al, 1975; Taylor and Watson, 1978; Swartz et al, 1986). It is indicated in the case of poor recipient area. In such cases we like to use microvascular bone grafts from the iliac crest or from the fibula to reconstruct the mandible in poor recipient areas of the midface. We use scapular bone grafts with a parascapular flap for the reconstruction of the maxilla and skin or mucosa (Hausamen and Schliephake, 1999b).[101]

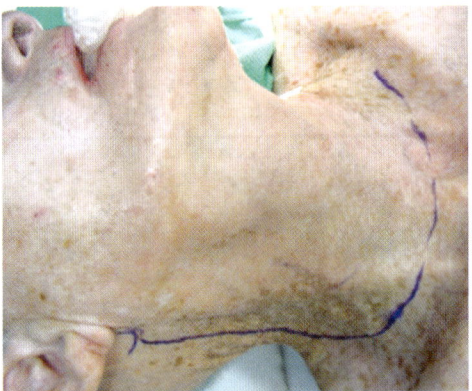 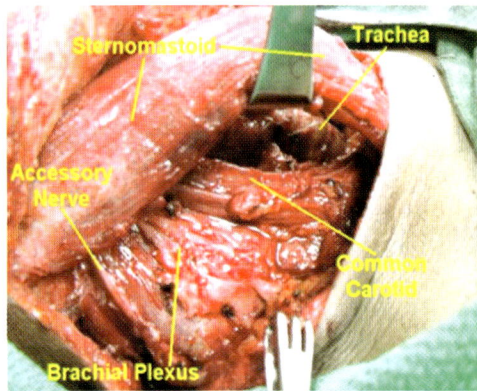

Fig. 5.2: A modified neck dissection in which **sternocleidomastoid is preserved.**

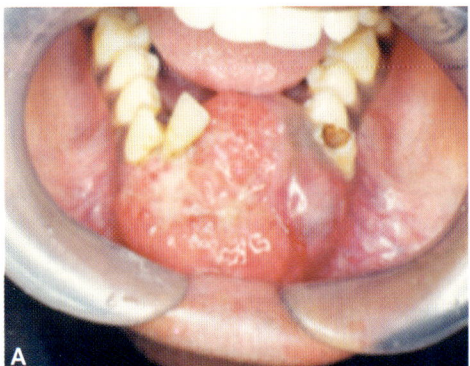 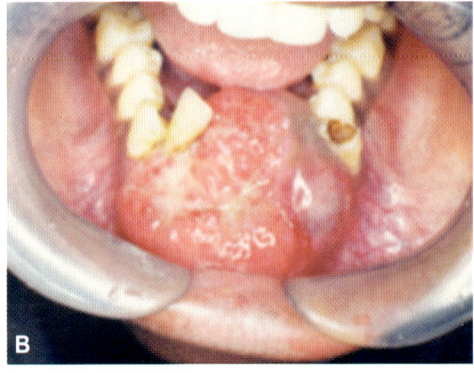

Preoperative intraoral view

Outline of extraoral incision for exposure

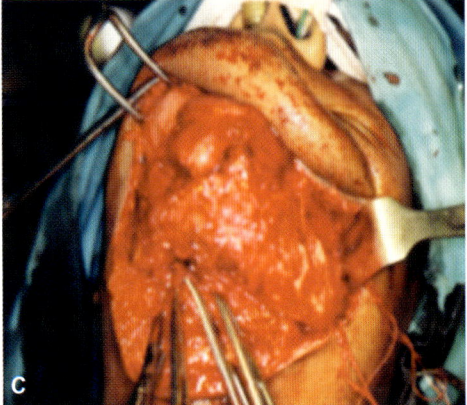 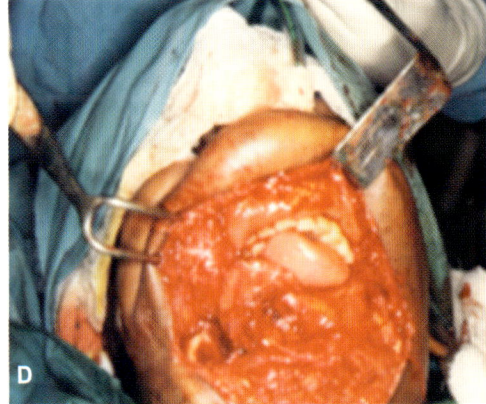

Tumor mass exposed by flap reflection and
dissection

Residual defect after excision of tumor mass

Figs 5.3A to D: Ablative surgery for resection of a tumor of mandible followed by reconstruction with a osteo-cutaneous microvascularised fibula graft

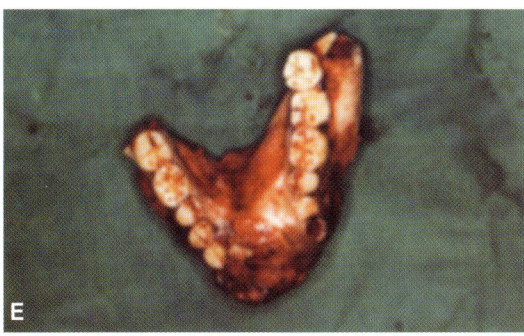

Specimen of tumor resected along with wide margin of dentoalveolar bone including the teeth

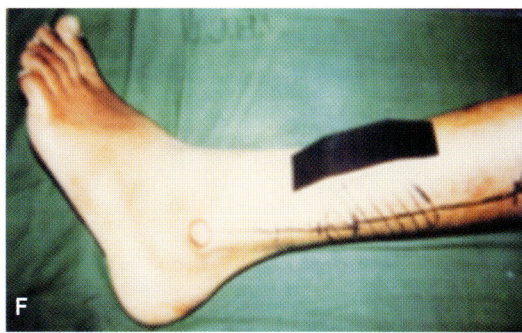

Planning done for resection of osteocutaneous fibula flap

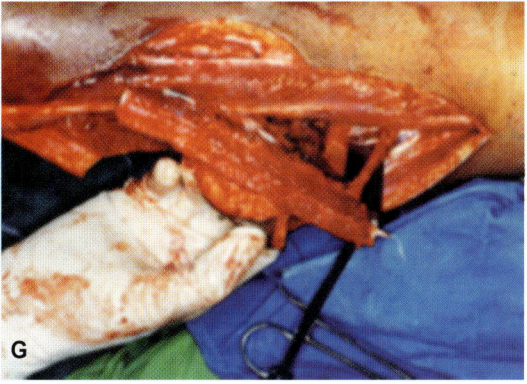

Graft dissected out along with the pedicle of peroneal artery

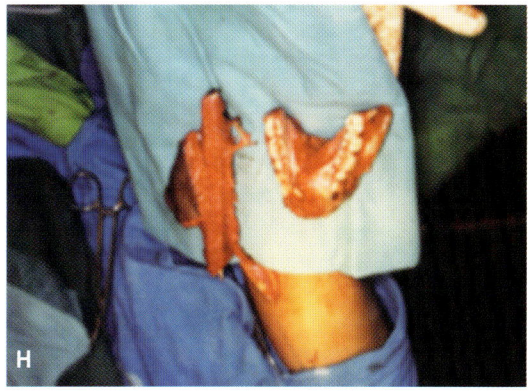

Comparison of resected specimen with the graft

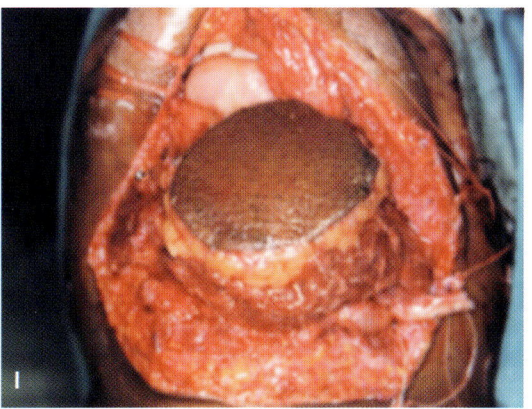

Microvascularised osteocutaneous fibula flap placed in the defect

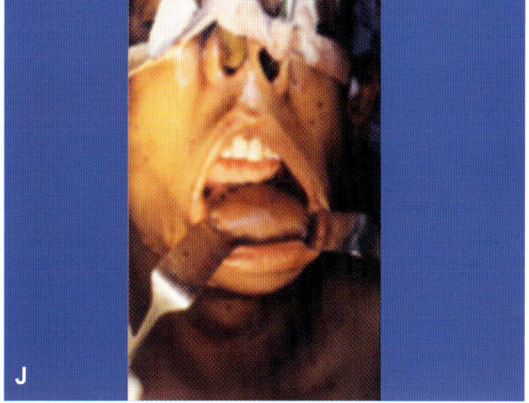

Immediate intraoral view after suturing.

Figs 5.3E to J: Ablative surgery for resection of a tumor of mandible followed by reconstruction with a osteocutaneous microvascularised fibula graft

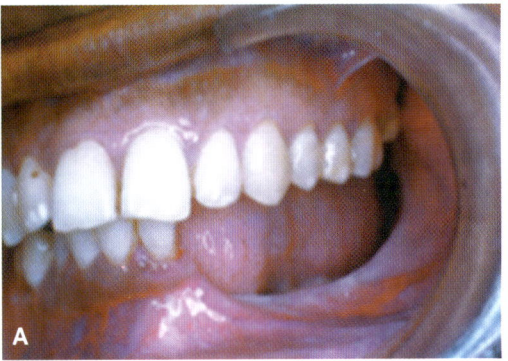

Preoperative intraoral view

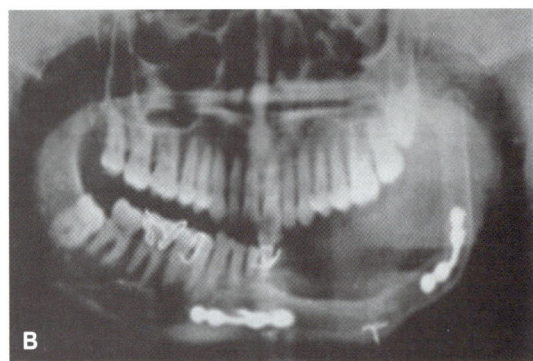

Preoperative OPG showing fixation of graft with miniplates

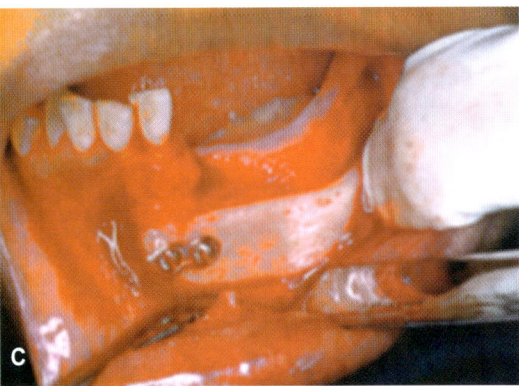

Exposure of graft after raising mucoperiosteal flap

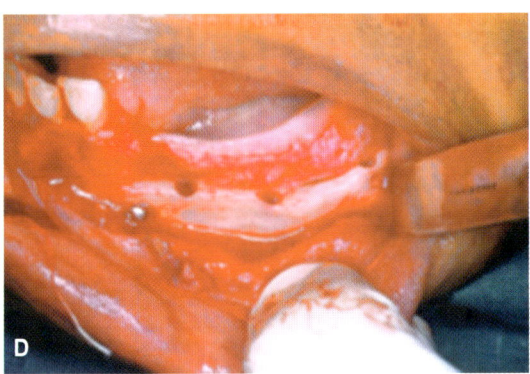

Graft prepared for implant placement

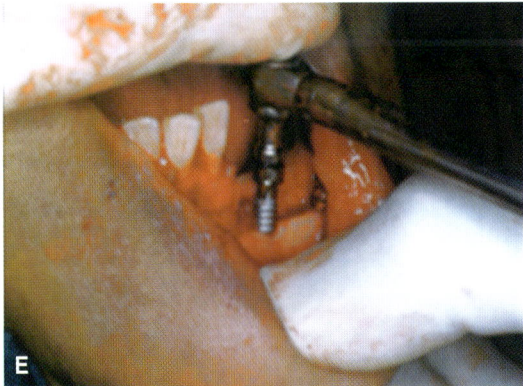

Implant being racheted in the prepared site of graft

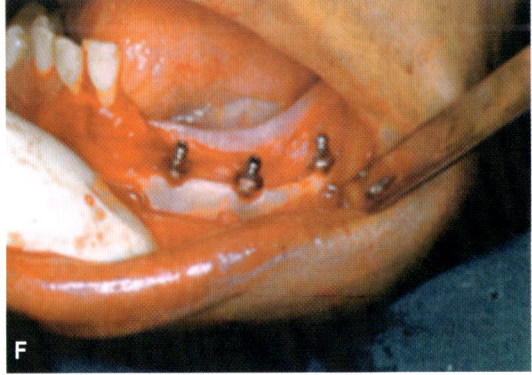

Three implants secured in place

Figs 5.4A to F: Oral rehabilitation of patient after reconstruction with microvascularised fibula graft.

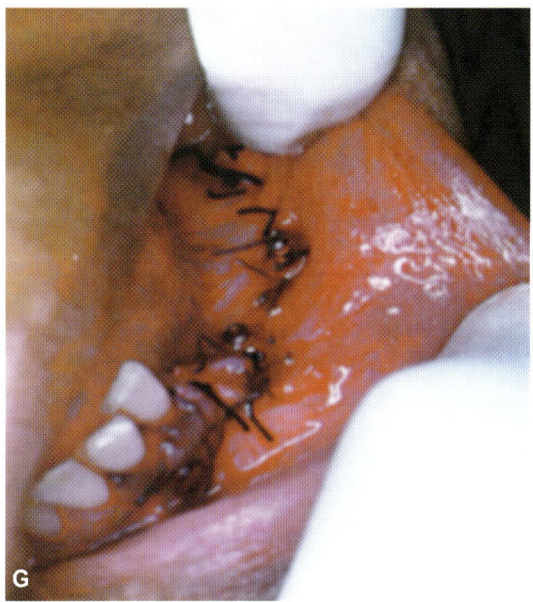

G

Flap closed

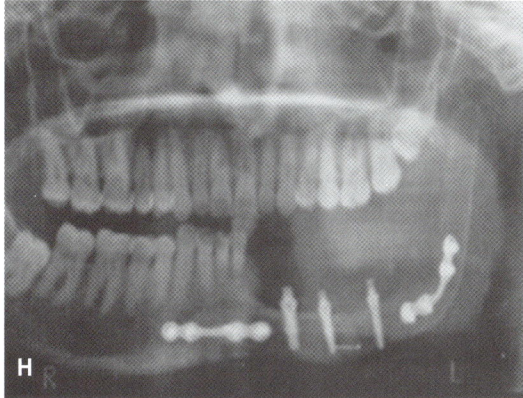

H

Postoperative OPG showing implant placement

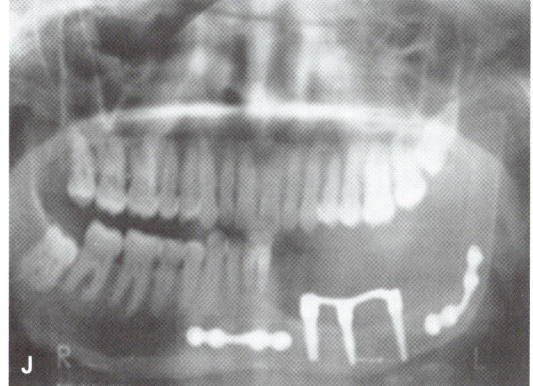

J

Postoperative OPG showing implants splinted with a casting bar

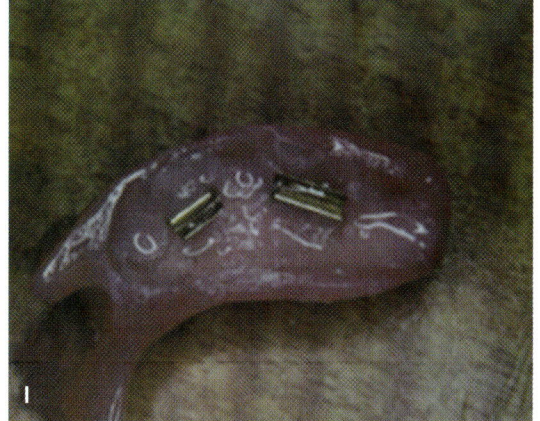

I

Tissue surface of prosthesis with metal attachments

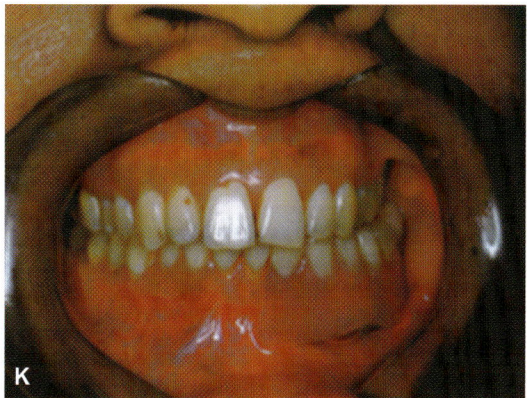

K

Implant supported prosthesis in place intraorally.

Figs 5.4G to K: Oral rehabilitation of patient after reconstruction with microvascularised fibula graft.

SKULL BASE ACCESS SURGERY

The base of the skull is a complex and relatively inaccessible region. Pathology in this area may arise from either within the skull itself or from adjacent areas such as the paranasal sinuses, the orbit and the face.

Conventional approaches to skull base lesions frequently require prolonged retraction of the brain and/or the resection of uninvolved structures to improve exposure. The resultant morbidity of such techniques, in terms of both cerebral function and facial appearance were often considerable with the result that many deep-seated skull based tumors were considered inoperable. The limited access also made adequate reconstruction of defects difficult and, in some cases, impossible.

Recent developments in surgical approaches to the skull base are based on the temporary disarticulation or dismantling of the skeleton of the face and the skull to varying degrees. These bone segments are mobilized either as free bone segments, completely detached from the soft tissues, or pedicled to the soft tissues to retain their blood supply. In most cases the so-called "access osteotomy" is combined with a conventional craniotomy. Facial incisions are avoided wherever possible—the coronal scalp flap and intraoral incisions providing adequate exposure in many cases.

If facial incisions are necessary, these are carefully sited and will usually heal with an imperceptible scar.

Maxillofacial surgeons, by virtue of their training in surgery of the facial bones and soft tissues, have contributed significantly to the development of the surgical access techniques now in common practice. The field of skull base surgery is developing rapidly. Sophisticated imaging techniques accurately identify both the position and dimensions of lesions and, in some cases, correctly diagnosing their nature.

Interventional radiologists can reduce the blood supply of tumors and vascular abnormalities further decreasing the potential morbidity of surgery, which at times allows surgeons to treat previously inoperable lesions.

The recent development of "navigation" systems enables surgeons to pinpoint their position in three dimensions at the time of surgery, which is of particular value where the pathology has destroyed the usual anatomical landmarks. The selective use of minimally invasive techniques and focused radiosurgery will also become more common as the limits of such techniques are appreciated. Notwithstanding these developments, adequate access to skull base pathology will remain an essential requirement for successful surgical treatment.[102]

IMAGE GUIDED NAVIGATION IN ORAL AND MAXILLOFACIAL SURGERY

Image-guided surgery is the logical extension of imaging as it integrates previously acquired radiological or nuclear medicine images with the operative field. In conventional image-guided surgery, a surgeon uses a surgical instrument or a pointer to establish correspondence between features in the preoperative images and the surgical scene. This is not ideal because the surgeon has to look away from the operative field to view the data.

Augmented reality guidance systems offer a solution to this problem but are limited by deformation of soft tissues. Real-time intraoperative imaging offers a potential solution but is currently only experimental. The additional precision and confidence that this technology provides make it a useful tool, and recent advances in image-guided surgery offer new opportunities in the field of oral and maxillofacial surgery.[103]

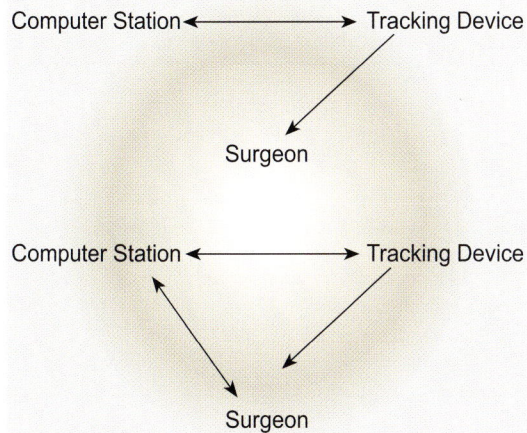

Fig. 5.5: Showing the comparison between conventional image guided surgery (upper) and augmented reality guided surgery (lower).

COMPUTERS IN OMFS

Advances in the basic scientific research within the field of computer assisted oral and maxillofacial surgery have enabled us to introduce features of these techniques into routine clinical practice. In order to simulate complex surgery with the aid of a computer, the diagnostic image data and especially various imaging modalities including computer tomography (CT), magnetic resonance imaging (MRI) and ultrasound (US) must be arranged in relation to each other, thus enabling a rapid switching between the various modalities as well as the viewing of superimposed images. Segmenting techniques for the reconstruction of three-dimensional representations of soft and hard tissues are required. This allows for a precise and fast entry of the planned surgical procedure in the planning and simulation phase. During the surgical phase, instrument navigation tools offer the surgeon interactive support through operation guidance and control of potential dangers. Future intraoperative assistance takes the form of such passive tools for the support of intraoperative orientation as well as so-called

'tracking systems' (semi-active systems) which accompany and support the surgeons' work. The final forms are robots that execute specific steps completely autonomously. The techniques of virtual reality and computer-assisted surgery are increasingly important in their medical applications. Many applications are still being developed or are still in the form of a prototype. It is already clear, however, that developments in this area will have a considerable effect on a surgeon's routine work.[104]

RADIOFREQUENCY IN ORAL AND MAXILLOFACIAL SURGERY

Radiofrequency surgery is a method of utilizing high frequency (3.8 to 4MHz) radiowave energy to incise, excise, or coagulate tissues. Radiofrequency (RF) is a relatively new modality that is being used for ano-rectal surgeries with increasing frequency. Radiofrequency energy consists of an alternating current that moves from an active electrode that is used within the area of treatment to dispersive electrodes that are placed on the patient. As the RF energy is applied, frictional heating of tissues results, with cell death occurring at temperatures between 60 and 1000° C.

Radiofrequency surgery has a lengthy documented **history** of use in oral, ophthalmic, plastic, and gynecology surgery. It was first used for the treatment of snoring. Gradually, its use in the practice of dermatology, cosmetology, cardiology, neurosurgery, hepatology, and ENT procedures gained momentum and popularity. It has multifaceted usages in the respective medical fields. However, there have been few published reports of its use in proctology. Radio surgery can simply be termed as an electro surgery at radiofrequency. The term 'radio' is used because the frequency of the device creating these waves is comparable to radiowave frequency used for broadcasting.

Electrocautery involves the passage of low frequency, low voltage, and low wattage alternating current (0.5–1.5 MHz) through the electrode, which resists the flow of current and becomes hot. In electrocautery, the heat [rather than the radio wave] is transferred to the soft tissue by convection. Massive cell destruction results from the application of cautery and the destruction caused by this cauterization are equivalent to that of a third degree burn.

While in hyfrecation, a highly modulated high frequency current of low wattage and high voltage is supplied to the electrode, and the surface of the tissue is burnt by a spark that is produced between the tip of the electrode and the tissue. Its effect is mainly superficial and it cannot be used to incise the tissue.

The high frequency radio surgery and its results should also not be confused with diathermy, electric cauterization, or spark producer. With radiofrequency, the targeted tissue temperatures stay localized within a 60–100° C range thus limiting heat dissipation and damage to adjacent tissue. In contrast, electrocautery, diathermy, or laser temperatures are significantly higher (750–900° C) which result in a very high heat propagation, which is far in excess of the desired therapeutic need.

Radiofrequency energy has been used extensively in many different medical applications and specialties for its ability to achieve a precise and controlled thermal ablation of soft tissue. The heat for this ablation is generated by a natural resistance of the tissue, which comes in the path of the waves released through the electrode tip of the device. The cellular water in the soft tissues gets heated and when the temperature reaches 100° C, it starts boiling and produces steam, which results in cellular molecular dissolution of individual tissue cells. The cells exposed to these waves are destroyed while the surrounding tissues remain unaffected. This property of radiofrequency eliminates the possibility of undue damage to the normal tissues, while improving the surgical precision.

The radiofrequency unit functions with the active electrode concentrating the high frequency energy at its tip, and then transmitting it to the passive electrode which returns the waves to the unit, making them more effective.

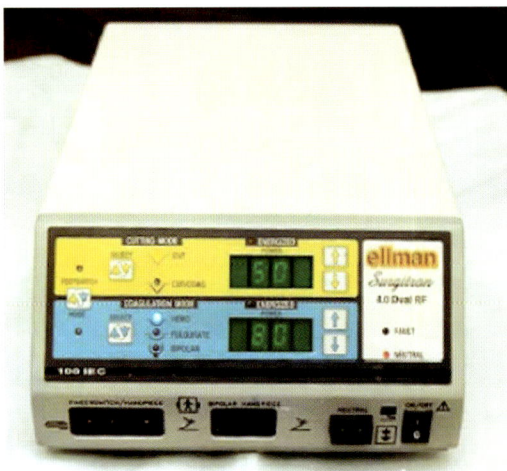

Fig. 5.6a: Radiofrequency unit

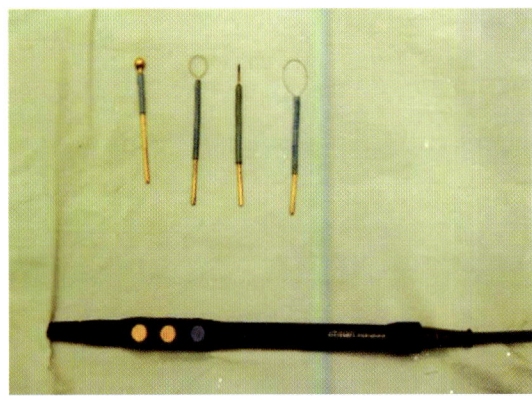

Fig. 5.6b: Hand piece and **electrodes**

PRECAUTIONS TO BE TAKEN WHILE OPERATING WITH THE RADIOFREQUENCY UNIT

Approximately ten seconds should be allowed for the tissues to cool between repeat applications of the electrodes. The two factors, which go to make this a good technique, involve the accuracy in power setting on the unit and the swift action of the cutting stroke.

Radiofrequency procedure should not be employed by, or on anyone who wears a pacemaker. The instrument should not be used in the presence of flammable or explosive liquids or gases. The skin under treatment should not be prepped with alcohol.

If proper settings are not known, the operator should start with a low power setting and cautiously increase power until an ideal cut is accomplished, without a tissue drag and no sparking. The finer the electrode used, the less would be the lateral heat spread and thus causing least damage to the adjacent tissues. It is recommended that a hands-on introductory course be taken before attempting the use of this technology.

Advantages

1. Allows cutting without pressure, and, consequently, there is little tissue damage and minimal scarring.
2. The electrode tip is sterile, as is all the tissue being exposed to it.
3. Healing is by granulation, with a soft and supple scar.
4. It could be with ease even in the depth and in difficult areas like the anal canal.
5. There are minimal incidences of postoperative infection, thereby achieving faster wound healing with negligible use of sutures, etc.[105]

Radiofrequency	Electrocautery
Requires different modes and adjustments	Simultaneous cut and coagulation
Minimal smoke production smoke.	Produces excessive
Minimal surrounding tissue damage.	Tissue damage like 3rd degree burns.
Heats tissues below 1000° C.	Raises tissue temperature above 500° C.
Sterilizes tissues under application.	Can cause postoperative sepsis.
Minimal scarring creates soft supple scar.	Gross scarring and fibrosis.
Faster healing.	Slow healing.

LASERS AND CRYOSURGERY

Both lasers and cryosurgery present a spectrum of exciting methods that result in a new concept of conservative surgery, augmentation and biomodulation. It is anticipated that they will find a special role in combination with gene therapy in the future, in relationship to orofacial malignant disease. Lasers lend themselves to gentle ablation of tissue with lack of bleeding and pain, while cryosurgery has special merits in relationship to nerve and bone that may regenerate after therapy. Both modalities of treatment are extremely important in the practice of oral and maxillofacial surgery.[106]

BOTOX IN COSMETIC FACIAL SURGERY

Wrinkling of facial soft tissues can lead to the appearance of aging that is easily noticed by our patients and their peers. Rejuvenation of some areas can be relatively straightforward and can lead to dramatic improvement of the maturing visage.

After one has evaluated the patient and arrived at a diagnosis, there are several office-based, outpatient procedures that can be utilized to correct the defect (s). Perhaps one of the simplest of these alternatives injection of *Clostridium botulinum* toxin type A to weaken forehead and periorbital depressor muscle contractions. This strategy can diminish wrinkles and frown lines and may even help to raise the brow superiorly. Use of this neurotoxin complex, alone or in combination with other materials and procedures, can provide a quick and facile method to improve facial cosmesis. Due to its neuromuscular blockade mechanism of action, botulinum toxin has found additional usefulness in the OMS office for the effective treatment of torticollis and masticatory musculature hyperactivity.[107]

MOLECULAR BIOLOGY AND ITS APPLICATIONS IN ORAL AND MAXILLOFACIAL SURGERY

Molecular biology is an exciting, rapidly expanding field, which has enabled enormously greater understanding of the biology of diseases and malfunctions in many fields. It chiefly concerns itself with understanding the interactions between the various systems of a cell, including the interrelationship of DNA, RNA and protein synthesis and how these interactions are regulated. Since the introduction of molecular biology into modern science, numerous other fields have been enabled to go "molecular". Advanced molecular biological techniques showed us new avenue towards finding answers to the questions asked for decades. It started as a joined discipline of other areas of biology, i.e. genetics and biochemistry in the 1930s and 1940s, and enjoyed its classical period and became institutionalized in the 1950s and 1960s. Major molecular techniques manipulating proteins, DNA and RNA were introduced and their mechanisms were concisely illustrated. The current knowledge of molecular biology and their applications in oral and maxillofacial surgery include bone fracture healing, oral cancer as well as craniofacial/dental anomalies and distraction osteogenesis. Although the problems of introducing molecular technologies are still substantial, it is anticipated that the future of medicine/dentistry will be "molecular": molecular prevention, molecular diagnosis and molecular therapy.[108]

GENE THERAPY

Modifications of traditional cancer therapies, including surgery, radiotherapy, and chemotherapy, have not improved the survival rates of patients with mucosal squamous cell carcinoma. Local and/or regional tumor recurrence develops in approximately one-third of patients, despite definitive treatment (Schwartz et al, 2000). The patient with recurrent or metastastic cancer is often considered incurable. A variety of chemotherapeutic agents have been used alone, and in combination, for the treatment of recurrent oral squamous cell carcinoma. However, chemotherapy is associated with well-known toxicities and has demonstrated no clear impact on survival in patients with recurrent oral cancer (Schrijvers et al, 1998).

Gene therapy has the potential to target cancer cells while sparing normal tissues. Such a strategy may be useful for recurrent disease as well as in the adjuvant setting (i.e., at the resected tumor margins). However, the clinical application of gene therapy for treatment of oral cancer will require optimization of gene delivery in conjunction with determinations of transfection efficiency.

Gene therapy can be defined as gene transfer for the purpose of treating human disease (Cusack and Tanabe, 1998). This includes the transfer of new genetic material as well as the manipulation of existing genetic material. This holds true especially for cancer cells, where dominantly activated oncogenes can be targeted. The transfer of genetic material may occur *in vivo* (where the gene is introduced into the body) or *ex vivo* (where a tumor is removed, the genetic materials delivered, and the cells are then re-introduced into the patient). The *ex vivo* approach has not been utilized in oral cancer because superficial lesions usually lend themselves to the direct injection of genetic material.

There are several general strategies utilized in a gene therapy approach to cancer, including:

1. Addition of a tumor-suppressor gene (gene addition therapy);

2. Deletion of a defective tumor gene (gene excision therapy);
3. Down-regulation of the expression of genes that stimulate tumor growth (antisense RNA);
4. Enhancement of immune surveillance (immunotherapy);
5. Activation of prodrugs that have a chemotherapeutic effect ("suicide" gene therapy);
6. Introduction of viruses that destroy tumor cells as part of the replication cycle;
7. Delivery of drug resistance gene(s) to normal tissue for protection from chemotherapy; and
8. Introduction of genes to inhibit tumor angiogenesis.

Genetic material can be transferred via a vector that is defined as the vehicle that is used to deliver the gene of interest. Chemical transfection introduces DNA by calcium phosphate, lipid, or protein complexes. Physical transfection of genes can be accomplished by electroporation, microinjection, or use of ballistic particles. Viruses commonly used in cancer gene therapies include retroviruses, adenoviruses, and herpes viruses. One limitation of retroviruses is that they can infect only actively dividing cells, leaving quiescent cells unaffected. However, the limitation of retroviral infection has been overcome, in part, by the use of lentiviral vectors, which have been shown to activate the immune system in pre-clinical animal models of oral cancer (Cardinali et al, 1998; Pang et al, 2001). Liposomes have no replication risk and are less immunogenic than viruses. The use of cationic liposomes as nonviral vehicles for the delivery of therapeutic molecules is becoming increasingly prevalent in the field of gene therapy. The transferrin ligand has been used to target a cationic liposome delivery system, resulting in a significant increase in the transfection efficiency of the complex (Xu et al, 1997).

GENE THERAPY STRATEGIES FOR ORAL CANCER

Gene Addition Therapy

Normal cells have the ability to regulate the cell cycle and eventually undergo programmed cell death (apoptosis). Cancer cells generally demonstrate impaired cell-cycle progression, largely due to mutations and overexpression of cell-cycle regulators (Gleich, 2000). The most extensively studied mutations in oral cancer are those of p53. Since the protein p53 plays a role in cell-cycle regulation and in apoptosis, p53 gene transfer was initially tested in squamous cell carcinoma patients by injecting the primary or regional tumor with an adenoviral vector expressing wild-type p53. Adenoviral p53 (Ad-p53) was demonstrated to be safe and well tolerated.

One of the primary challenges in efforts to introduce tumor suppressor genes is the transfection of all target cells. The required transfection efficiency to elicit an anti-tumor response is generally unknown, although one could logically predict that the most efficacious treatment would be delivered to the highest proportion of target cells.

ANTISENSE RNA AND RIBOZYMES

Gene expression can usually be inhibited by RNA that is complementary to the strand of DNA expressing the gene. This "antisense" RNA can prevent the activity of several known oncogenes, including myc, fos, and ras, and can inhibit viruses such as HSV-1, HPV, and HTLV-1 (Wickstrom et al, 1988; Maeda et al, 1998). Such therapy can theoretically be directed toward carcinoma cells whose malignant phenotype is dependent upon the expression of particular oncogenes. Inhibition of expression of these oncogenes may alter the phenotype, thus abrogating tumor growth.

Inhibition of tumor growth in xenograft models of oral cancer is recently observed with

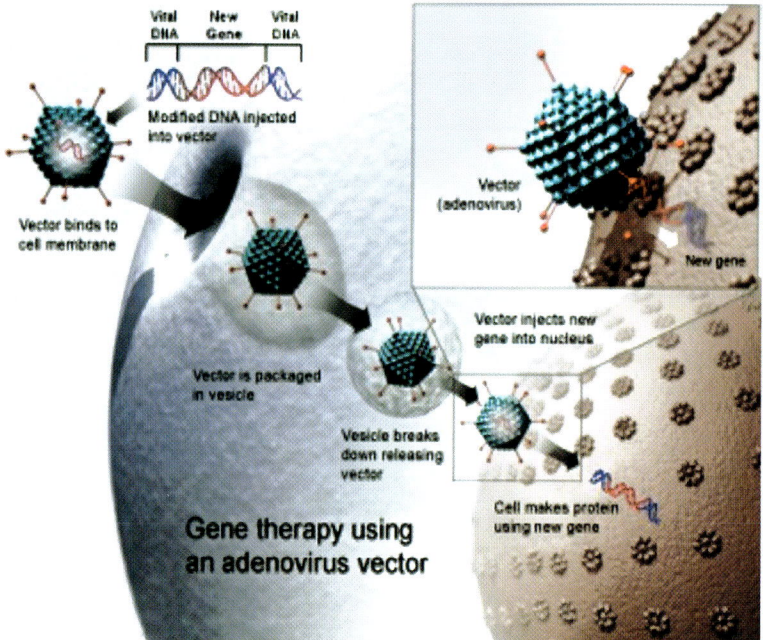

Fig. 5.7: A new gene is injected into an adenovirus vector, which is used to introduce the modified DNA into a human cell. If the treatment is successful, the new gene will make a functional protein

systemic administration of EGFR antisense DNA (unpublished observations). The ability of gene-specific double-stranded RNA to trigger the degradation of homologous cellular RNAs is known as RNA interference (RNAi). Small interfering RNAs (siRNAs) mediate mRNA degradation in the process of RNAi and have been shown in recent studies to be potentially more effective than antisense RNA, likely due to enhanced resistance of siRNAs to nuclease degradation (Bertrand et al, 2002).

IMMUNOTHERAPY

The immunologic gene therapy approach to oral cancer involves either increasing the immunogenic potential of tumor cells or augmenting the patient's immune response to a tumor. Patients with squamous cell carcinoma of the head and neck demonstrate deficient function of several categories of immune cells, including natural killer cells, T-lymphocytes,

and several cytokines (Gleich, 2000). Although oral cancer is not classically immunogenic, there is abundant evidence for immune recognition. The feasibility and efficacy of combination non-viral lipid-formulated murine interleukin 2 (mIL-2) and polymer-formulated murine interleukin 12 (mIL-12) gene therapy for squamous cell carcinoma has been investigated in pre-clinical models. The use of combined mIL-2 and mIL-12 gene therapy resulted in significant anti-tumor effects, most likely due to increased activation of cytolytic T lymphocyte and natural killer cells (Li et al, 2001).

"SUICIDE" GENE THERAPY

"Suicide" gene therapy involves the introduction of a gene into a cell that enables a prodrug to be activated into an active cytotoxic drug. The most extensively studied approach utilizes Herpes Simplex Virus-Thymidine.

Kinase (HSV-TK). This gene encodes a viral enzyme that phosphorylates ganciclovir into a monophosphate form, which is then further phosphorylated by intracellular enzymes into an active triphosphate compound that terminates DNA synthesis (Matthews and Boehme, 1988). Thus, this system selectively targets actively dividing cancer cells.

REPLICATING VIRUSES THAT DESTROY TUMOR CELLS

A novel approach to gene therapy that has been extensively evaluated in pre-clinical and clinical studies for squamous cell carcinoma involves a vector that selectively replicates within and lyses tumor cells. An E1B 55kD gene-deleted adenovirus, ONYX-015 (d11520), has been developed for the treatment of tumors lacking p53 function (Heise et al, 1999). ONYX-015 can be safely administered via intra-tumoral injection to patients with recurrent/refractory squamous cell carcinoma. However, evidence of only modest anti-tumoral activity has been detected when this approach to gene therapy was used alone (Kirn et al, 1998; Nemunaitis et al, 2001).[109]

ADVANCES IN DISTRACTION TECHNIQUES FOR CRANIOFACIAL SURGERY

Distraction osteogenesis has been applied to the craniofacial skeleton as well as the long bones of the extremities. This technique does not require bone grafting and allows correction of craniofacial deformities with less invasion. Moreover, the distraction procedures can expand the overlying soft tissues simultaneously. Administration of some cytokines for shortening the consolidation period may be considered. Among disorders indicated for distraction osteogenesis, there are several syndromic craniosynostoses, which involve mutations in the fibroblast growth factor receptor (FGFR) 2 gene. The FGFR 2 mutation was suggested to clinically accelerate osteogenesis at the distraction site.

The usefulness and appropriateness of the distraction protocol must be assessed for each individual disorder. Although distraction osteogenesis in the craniofacial skeleton has advanced technologically, all possible risks must be discussed, especially until establishment of fully safe distraction procedures.[110]

REFERENCES AND BIBLIOGRAPHY

97. Editorial of J Oral Maxillofacial Surg 62:1–2, 2004.
98, 99, 100, 101 "The scientific development of maxillofacial surgery in the 20th century and an outlook into the future" — article from Journal of Craniomaxillofacial surgery: 2001; Feb29 (1); Pg 2–21.
102, 106. History of British Association of Oral and Maxillofacial Surgery from the web.
103. Image guided navigation—British Journal of Oral and Maxillofacial Surgery (2005); 43:294–302.
104. Computer assisted oral and maxillofacial surgery—a review and an assessment of technology —Int J Oral Maxillofac Surg 2001; 30: 2–13.
105. From the web "Radiofrequency surgery: offering a novel approach to ano-rectal diseases"—Middle East Journal of Family Medicine, 2005; Vol. 3 (1).
107. Botox : Cosmetic and Functional Uses in Oral and Maxillofacial Surgery—Steven A. Guttenberg, DDS, MD, Washington, DC—American Society for Aesthetic Plastic Surgery: Member Practice Profile 2003.
   References: Garcia, Fulton: Botox response v. dosage. Dermatol Surg 22:39, 1996 Carruthers A, Carruthers J, Said S: Double-blind, randomized, parallel group, dose-ranging study of botulinum toxin type A in the treatment of glabellar lines. Division of Dermatology, University of British Columbia, Vancouver, BC, Canada.
108. "Molecular biology and its applications in orthodontics and oral and maxillofacial surgery".—article from : Shanghai Kou Qiang Yi Xue. 2005 Jun; 14(3): 311–8.
109. Gene therapy –"Gene Therapy For The Treatment of Oral Squamous Cell Carcinoma" taken from Article of J Dent Res 82(1): 11-16, 2003.
110. "Advances in distraction techniques for craniofacial surgery"—article from J Med Invest. 2003 Aug; 50(3-4):117–25.

Chapter **6**

Future Prospects in Oral and Maxillofacial Surgery

First of all there is the basic question whether classical surgery as we know it today will actually survive in the years to come: the rapid new developments in the field of medical technology, the introduction of microrobots, minimal invasive and laser surgery jeopardizing the classic role of the surgeon. He is being replaced by computers and other technological devices. The rapid growth of gene technology also may render the indication for surgery superfluous in many cases so far requiring surgery.

But how about oral and cranio-maxillofacial surgery in the years to come!! Dental problems calling for surgical intervention have existed from the very beginning of mankind until today. The raison d'etre (the most important reason for existence) for oral surgery will not be jeopardized for many years. However, the major dental diseases such as caries and periodontal disease, will be mastered in the near future, so that the field of oral surgery in the Western countries will change and include more and more restorative measures. Most likely we will not be able to cope with the consequences of physiological aging in the near future so that more and more elderly people will ask for functional dental replacement. In

this respect, implatotology offers favourable prospects. While the insertion of implants into local bone is a safe routine method today, the treatment of an atrophic jaw or traumatically induced jaw defects is still presenting many problems. These problems will be solved in the near future without the grafting of autogenous bone as done today.

With regard to the future development of the treatment of clefts, there may be new concepts every now and then, although we have already reached a high standard in cleft treatment. Today it is still difficult to say whether new developments in prenatal diagnostics and new anaesthesiological and surgical techniques in fetal surgery will receive much clinical attention or not. So far animal experiments and first clinical results of prenatal surgery in human fetuses have suggested that intrauterine surgery of cleft lips could be feasible. It would have the advantage of favorable fetal wound healing, However, so far we do not have any clinical experience with those new methods and for the time being we are very hesitant to apply them because of ethical reasons.

Today the surgical techniques of moving the bones of the skull have reached certain perfection and are standardized. However, distraction osteogenesis may be applied even more frequently in the near future. The use of navigation systems and operating robots has not fully been accepted yet, although they would mean increased accuracy in the planning and performance of osteotomies. It also seems likely to prevent recurrences by using intraoperative fixation including a more accurate positioning of the condyle. Further developments in the field of computer-aided simulation will probably make available new systems of three-dimensional imaging helping in the planning of cranio-maxillofacial surgery by simulating all aspects of the bony segments to be repositioned and imaging the consequent changes in the soft tissue at the same time (Reuther, 2000).

Other fields of maxillofacial surgery, however, will experience a more serious change: the results of basic research will deeply affect our operating techniques. For the next few years, we cannot imagine any quantum leaps in tumor surgery comparable to the introduction of myocutaneous flaps or microsurgery. We do not expect any important progress in the traditional field of surgery (Hausamen and Schliephake, 1999a).

In cranio-maxillofacial surgery today, (it can be thought that) we have reached the peak of radical tumor resection. We will concentrate increasingly our efforts on saving structures. We will also concentrate on reconstructing and repairing structures, and we will succeed in restoring not only the anatomy, as is possible today, but also the function of tissues in large defects. This is in context with the difficult reconstruction of the tongue and restoration of its function which is so extremely important for the quality of life and rehabilitation of our patients. Perhaps the transplantation of an entire allogenic tongue could meet the requirements of full restitutio ad integrum. For the time being, such a procedure is contraindicated because of the negative side effects of immunosuppression and the unsolved

problem of a possible virus infection from the transplanted organ (Hausamen et al, 1994).

The new developments in tumor therapy will be in a totally different field. New perspectives resulting from basic research, especially in molecular biology can be expected. In the past 20 years molecular biology has already provided a lot of important information on oncogenesis, on how and why tumors develop. This has resulted in new theories on the prevention, diagnosis and therapy of tumors some of which are already being applied in the clinical routine today. Cells, molecules and genes, and not organs are in the center of oncological research nowadays, whose function within an organism are explained and whose functional or structural deficiencies can be influenced by means of recombination gene technology.

The future results of molecular biology regarding the origin and development of a tumor disease will have an effect on the surgical methods of tumor therapy, and the question arises whether we will be able to do without surgery altogether. If molecular biology will make the great breakthrough in medicine, it may be that tumor surgery will disappear from our operating rooms in the long run. Gene therapy represents a new and innovative approach to the treatment of cancer, including oral cancer. As our understanding of the molecular mechanisms of cancer increases, it is possible to exploit these principles and to target tumor cells selectively.

We will also experience new developments in the field or tissue transplantation, which by the way is so closely connected with tumor therapy. The grafts harvested for bridging large defects are characterized by a high rate of perioperative morbidity. Therefore several attempts are being made to do without harvesting autogenous grafts and to produce the graft at that place where it is required. Regarding autogenous bone grafting which is still considered the gold standard of bone grafting, research in the field of osteoconduction and osteoinduction is leading into a new direction. The biological mechanisms of osteoconduction and osteoinduction arc largely known today and we are presently on the threshold from experimental to clinical studies (Urist et al, 1983; Kubler et al, 1991; 1995, 1998; Schliephake et al, 1996, 1997, 1998).

While osteoconduction is using the regenerative capacity of local bone by providing a suitable structure, the mechanism of osteoinduction is characterized by the differentiation of pluripotent mesenchymal cells in good recipient areas into cartilage-forming and bone-forming precursor cells under the influence of morphogenetic proteins. Our present understanding of the biomechanical mechanism of the particular protein fraction called bone morphogenetic proteins (BMP) is already very good. Nine different types of BMPs have been isolated so far and it has been possible to produce them using gene technology. Thus it is not an unrealistic dream that in the near future new bone will be formed not only at the location of the defect, but also away from the defect and that such bone is then transplanted to the maxillofacial region by a suitable carrier substance. (Schliephake and Langner, 1997; Schliephake and Aleyt, 1998; Terheyden et al, 1999). Similar research is being done on the creation of cartilage, skin and mucosa. 'Tissue engineering' is the term for all these new methods.

The two examples of osteoconduction and osteoinduction which could be supplemented by research in other special fields, show that in cranio-maxillofacial surgery again and again new therapeutical methods will arise which will replace some of our traditional surgical techniques and at the same time widen and increase our therapeutic facilities.

The spectrum of cranio-maxillofacial surgery will grow in the next years; it will become more and more complex. Expertly trained maxillofacial surgeons, well equipped and well funded research centers and universities as well as the implementation of a research policy oriented towards the future will be needed to cope with the new challenges.

The older generation of maxillofacial surgeons is asked to inspire the young maxillofacial surgeons and arouse their curiosity so that they can meet the future challenges with enthusiasm and understand them as a great chance. We have to provide a good scientific and clinical foundation for our young colleagues so that equipped with additional knowledge in business management, computer technology, medical ethics and medical politics, they are able to find their way in the future media world. On the basis of a good knowledge of basic research, improved technical facilities and unlimited possibilities of information, they will need curiosity and enthusiasm to meet the challenges of the new century.

The field of crania-maxillofacial surgery will change; it will be necessary to develop new concepts of identification and self-understanding. They will be based on the standards established by our generation of maxillofacial surgeons. The following generation will formulate new targets, develop new fascinating goals and will successfully reach them.

To conclude it is worth mentioning regarding the world fair at New York. At the New York World's fair, the General Motors exhibit showed a future of sleek vehicles moving seamlessly on rivers of concrete towards glorious cities reaching for the sky. The reality of that vision can be seen in the concretion of steel immobilized in today's sprawling cities.[111]

REFERENCES AND BIBLIOGRAPHY

111. "The scientific development of maxillofacial surgery in the 20th century and an outlook into the future"—article from Journal of Craniomaxillofacial surgery: 2001; Feb 29 (1);2-21.

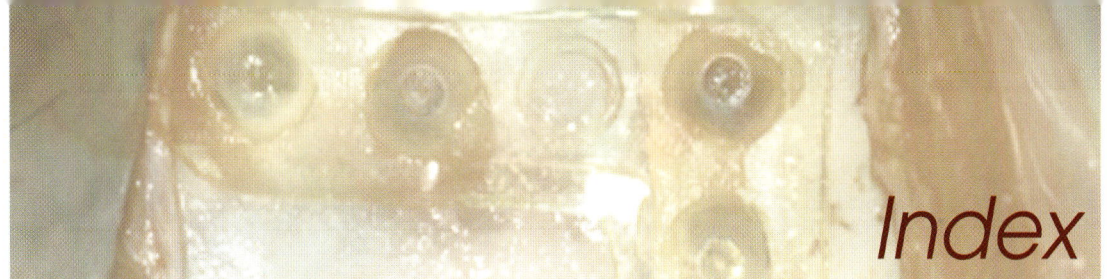

Index